Midwife on Call

Tales of Tiny Miracles

AGNES LIGHT

Midwife on Call

Tales of Tiny Miracles

HODDER

First published in Great Britain in 2011 by Hodder & Stoughton
An Hachette UK company

1

ISBN 978 1 444 73612 0
eBook ISBN 978 1 444 73613 7

Typeset in Sabon by Hewer Text UK Ltd, Edinburgh

Printed and bound in the UK by CPI Mackays, Chatham ME5 8TD

Hodder & Stoughton policy is to use papers that are natural, renewable and recyclable products and made from wood grown in sustainable forests. The logging and manufacturing processes are expected to conform to the environmental regulations of the country of origin.

Hodder & Stoughton Ltd
338 Euston Road
London NW1 3BH

www.hodder.co.uk

In memory of Penny Littleford

November 18th 1957 – September 28th 2010

For my children and grandchildren

Contents

1

Starting Out

'Come on, love, push now!' coaxed the midwife. (How familiar those words were to become – over more than thirty years of my career as a midwife, I must have used them myself thousands of times!)

'I am bloody pushing!' grunted the red-faced woman propped up on the bed. She had already been in labour for eight hours and was entering the second stage, which is the moment when things can get really desperate, when the woman can begin to fear that the pain might never end, and the baby might never come. Standing next to the bed was a terrified young man who was about to become a father for the first time. I shot him a reassuring smile, but he was clearly too nervous to take any notice.

As if she wasn't already going through enough, the woman in labour had an audience. In one corner of that cramped little room stood six of us girls: an ill-assorted bunch, also waiting for the arrival of the baby. It was the very first day of our midwifery training. We can hardly have been a reassuring sight to the poor parents-to-be. We wore paper hats like shower caps to cover our hair and masks to cover our faces. In fact, if we hadn't been so scared, we probably would have laughed at the sight of each other.

We were all gathered in a room in an old teaching hospital. We'd barely had time to get acquainted, and now here we were attending one of the most intimate and emotional events in a woman's life. I glanced nervously at the other girls . . . was I the only one feeling so hot? My skin was prickling and my hands were sweating. I dug my nails into my palms and tried to pull myself together. Even though I'd had two babies myself, I hadn't seen events from this position. It brought back so many memories of my own experience of childbirth: how terrifying and overwhelming it had been the first time, how much I had needed the comfort and expertise of the midwife, who had been through this process hundreds of times with other women. I knew what this poor woman was going through because I had been there myself. I willed her to stay calm and to concentrate on what the midwife was telling her. 'Now pant, don't push. You're nearly there; the baby's nearly here . . .'

As I watched the little head emerging, the light overhead seemed to grow brighter. The woman's groans and the midwife's voice faded into the distance and my head began to swim. Sensing that I was going to faint, I stumbled to the door and, once outside, collapsed gratefully onto a conveniently placed chair, lowering my head between my knees. Oh dear! Everybody makes jokes about fathers passing out at births, but surely midwives don't faint? Well, they're certainly not supposed to, anyway. How would I ever make the grade?

As I tried to collect myself, taking long deep breaths, several midwives passed me in the corridor, some looking sympathetic, others giggling at me. Suddenly our tutor appeared and ushered me back into the room, like a mother hen herding a stray chick.

'You must come and see the placenta being delivered now!'

I knew I needed to get back in there – this is one of the most important stages of the delivery process, and I wanted to observe it – but part of me was worried I'd keel over in front of the poor woman. Anyway, my tutor didn't give me any choice, and thankfully I managed to stay upright, despite all the blood. I had never seen so much. And of course when I went back in, the atmosphere in the room had changed completely. The baby had arrived safe and well, and suddenly all the pain and anxiety were swept away. All of the student midwives were grinning and relaxed, and I remember looking in awe at the senior midwife who had caught this gorgeous new baby in her hands and handed him to his mother for the very first time. She seemed totally calm. She smiled back at me when I gave her a nervy grin, very embarrassed about my fainting episode, and just got on with the cleaning-up process.

Luckily the parents were totally oblivious to my comings and goings; they were so delighted with their new baby. I was amazed they hadn't objected to the presence of six peering onlookers in the first place, but perhaps they hadn't been consulted. After all, this was 1976 and the medicalisation of childbirth was in full swing. Patients' feelings weren't necessarily top priority.

Our tutor was quite kind to me that day. She understood that watching the delivery had probably brought back memories of the births of my own children, who were six and seven years old at the time. My recollection of childbirth was so powerfully emotional that I fainted again at the next few births I attended. It got to the point where a chair was always placed outside any delivery room in which I happened to be. One tutor used to get quite impatient with me. 'You'll never become a midwife!' she scolded.

But I'm glad to say I proved her wrong. Despite my funny turn that day, I never forgot the joy on those parents' faces when they held their child for the first time. Before we all trooped out of the room, I heard the new mother say, 'Thank you for everything,' to the midwife who had helped her. When I turned round on my way out I saw the look that passed between the two of them. Mutual respect and a deep sense of comfort and gratitude. 'It was a pleasure, love,' the midwife said warmly. In that moment I vowed that this was something I would do, and do well.

And so our training had begun. None of us were qualified nurses already. However, we had all decided that midwifery was to be our chosen profession and we were lucky enough to be accepted on a two-year fast-track course.

We were all from very different backgrounds. Two of the girls were nursery nurses, one worked in local government, another had been an air hostess and one was a personal assistant.

My background was different again.

I grew up in a loving home in a commuter town in Kent. I was the middle of three children; my father ran a flooring business and my mother didn't work when we were young; she stayed at home with us. In many ways, mine was a typical 1950s childhood, happy and innocent, although there were problems beneath the surface caused by my father's moodiness, which I later came to understand was triggered by his alcoholism. It was a time when people didn't discuss their feelings and problems anywhere near as openly as they do now and my parents were very old-fashioned in outlook, so there was a lot that was swept under the carpet. For instance, no-one ever mentioned sex or what lay behind my father's mood swings.

Ever since I'd been a small child I had wanted to be a nurse. I remember bandaging my father up and tending to imaginary wounds on his body while he was sitting relaxing in the evenings. And I watched *Emergency Ward 10* and *Dr. Kildare* on the television religiously in the 1950s and 60s. I never considered any other career. My parents encouraged me. They very much wanted me to make something of myself. I know my mother wanted me to have a worthwhile career.

After leaving school I completed a one-year secretarial course, mainly to please my mother. I didn't enjoy it much, although looking back I wish I had learnt to touch-type, as it would have been very useful in this computer-driven age. Instead I joked around with the girls in my class and only put in the minimum of effort, because I didn't think I would ever need secretarial skills.

After my secretarial course and a spell working for a youth employment service, I was lucky enough to be accepted at University College Hospital in London to start my training. In 1967 five O levels were required and I had managed to acquire seven, despite not being a particularly diligent student. The headmistress of my grammar school spoke to my parents about me one day.

'She really should consider medicine as a career, not nursing,' she pronounced. I suppose this was quite forward-thinking of her in the 1960s, when as a matter of course boys became doctors and girls nurses. But I wouldn't even contemplate medicine. My heart was set on nursing and it always had been.

When I was a little girl, I wanted to be a children's nurse. I've always adored children: my brother was born when I was nine years old and I loved cuddling him and playing with him. Then as time went on, I had it in my mind that I'd like to become a midwife. This was partly because I had a cousin who was a midwife and she was always telling me about her work. But I think my fascination with my mother's pregnancy might also have had something to do with it. It amazed me to see her belly expanding and to think that there was a baby growing inside her; it was even more incredible when the baby came along one day! My brother's birth seemed like a miracle, especially since my mother didn't talk much about her pregnancy. That generation just didn't. Mum was a very caring, nurturing person who loved babies and children, but she wouldn't even say the word pregnant; 'expecting' was as far as she would go. I think she may also have been a bit embarrassed about being a mum-to-be again at the age of forty-three, which was considered ancient to be having a baby in those days, and perhaps even a little unseemly.

When I was eighteen, before the rules changed, you had to qualify as a nurse before you became a midwife. So my nurse's training was my primary focus when I embarked on my career. I felt so proud the day I heard that I'd been accepted onto the nursing course. I'd been very nervous at the interview and thought I might have ruined everything. I knew I was qualified academically, but of course a large part of being a good nurse is having the ability to get on with people, to be calm and kind and interested in what vulnerable people need and want. I worried that maybe I hadn't seemed self-possessed enough, but I suppose the interviewer must have been used to seeing terrified young girls because she passed me.

Everyone in my family shared my excitement, especially my grandmother, who had wanted to be a nurse many decades before but had been unable to fulfil her dream. I loved my grandmother to bits; she was like a second mum to me. She lived close by and as my grandfather died before we were born, she focused all her love and attention on us. I know she was a huge help to my mother when my brother was little. That's something that I have seen get lost over the course of my career: the involvement of extended family in caring for women in the immediate aftermath of childbirth, and for their children. Certainly I was very close to my gran. You have a different relationship with your grandparents, don't you? They're much more indulgent than your parents and you can get away with so much more! I often went to stay with my grandmother as a child and now that she was old and becoming increasingly frail, she had come to live with us. We often talked about what lay ahead for me in my nurse's training; she wanted to hear all about what my course would entail and where I'd be living.

I was aware that Gran was in decline, but that didn't prepare me for her death just before I started my training. I was completely grief-stricken; an aching hole opened up in me and I found it very hard to come to terms with the loss of such an important person in my life. It was my first encounter with mortality and I found it very shocking. Part of me knew that at least my gran had lived a full life, and had been cherished by her family right up until the end, but I was also reeling from the experience of bereavement. It simply felt too big to deal with.

At the same time, it was a huge thrill to begin my new career, and I knew that Gran would have been so proud of me as I set off on my first day, so I tried my best to put my sadness aside and make the most of the moment.

The hospital was in the centre of London in a very grand, old building, and the training school was attached to it. Although it was old, the architecture was beautiful and imposing and I felt so excited to be there. It made me very proud the first time I put on the hospital uniform, which comprised a stiff grey dress with separate little white cuffs for the sleeves and a starched white pinafore apron. There was also a rather complicated starched cap which started off as a flat stiff square of white cotton and ended up like a little meringue with a frill perched on top of the head. The whole ensemble was finished off with black stockings and suspenders, which may be a turn-on for some men but were actually very uncomfortable to wear! It took quite a long time to get ready in the mornings and, to be honest, the outfit was not really suited to the job in hand.

The first eight weeks of training were spent entirely in the classroom, learning the basics of anatomy, physiology, health and sickness, as well as the practical skills such as blanket-bathing. This had always been a rather mysterious term to me as I had no idea what went on underneath the blanket. I soon found out, of course.

I loved the training; I loved living away from home for the first time and the camaraderie that developed among my fellow students. The whole experience was exactly as I had always dreamed it would be. I felt successful and independent and so thrilled that I was making good on my long-held ambition. I had been looking forward to being a nurse for as long as I could remember, I had invested so much determination and longing, and it could so easily have turned out to be a disappointment. But to my delight, it was every bit as good as I'd thought it would be.

The only thing I didn't like was being away from my boyfriend back home. It was my first serious romance: John was my first lover and the man I hoped to marry. I travelled home from London most weekends to be with him. In those days men were not allowed in the students' rooms at the nurses' home and we had to be indoors at ten o'clock at night. Even though this was the Swinging Sixties, the nursing profession was still rather Victorian in outlook. Naturally we managed to find ways around these rules: we were teenagers after all! At one entrance to the hospital there was an underground tunnel which led to the nurses' home, and we always used it to avoid getting caught returning home late.

When I started working on the wards it was even more exciting, but terrifying too. It was a real challenge to face serious illness and death on a daily basis at the age of eighteen, especially when I was feeling so raw from my own bereavement. The patients and their relatives were usually older than me, yet they were strangers who were vulnerable and needed help and kindness. Trying to support them through terminal illness and death was really difficult at that age. You had people saying to you, 'Am I going to die?' and you'd be thinking, 'I'm eighteen! I don't know what to say.' It made us all grow up very quickly. I had a lot of empathy for people because of losing my grandmother, but I don't know whether that made it harder or easier overall. I found it awkward to talk about her, because it made me cry, and so I didn't always manage to get across the fact that I knew how the patients and their families felt.

Doing intimate things for the older patients was also very daunting. One admission to the ward during my first week was a man who had fallen from scaffolding; both of his arms were encased in plaster, rendering them useless. I vividly remember the awful sinking feeling I experienced when he called me over to say he needed to pass urine and indicated the bottle for this purpose sitting on his locker. It was obvious that he couldn't use the bottle without help, but what was I supposed to do? I hurried over to the staff nurse to ask her advice.

'You have to pick his "manhood" up and put it in the bottle for him, of course, Nurse!' she said, giving me a withering look.

So that's what I did. I managed it, but only with great embarrassment, as I wasn't yet used to nonchalantly handling strangers' body parts!

It didn't take me long to realise that I had led a fairly sheltered life. One day, a male patient was admitted to the ward haemorrhaging from the anus and in urgent need of a blood transfusion. The ward sister gave the nurses a report about him, as was customary.

'This gentleman has been damaged by his friend,' she said enigmatically.

When I questioned one of the senior nurses about it later, she enlightened me. 'The man is a homosexual and he bled heavily from the rectum after anal intercourse.'

I was so shocked that I couldn't speak! Until then, I'd had no idea of what gay people did during sex. This was the start of my education about real life and we students spent many hours exchanging lurid tales of what we had seen, done and heard on the wards. I think we were all in the same boat when it came to being quite immature and naive, and we'd rush to each other's rooms to talk about all these strange and terrible things. Sometimes our tales were funny and sometimes they were sad – and we comforted and supported each other through all the traumas. We also had a lot of fun discussing the hunky doctors and medical students. After all, it was virtually every student nurse's dream to marry a doctor – whether or not she had a boyfriend back home!

There were a few girls I was very friendly with: Geri, who was a doctor's daughter and very well educated; Debbie, who was always there to listen when you had a problem; and Barbara, a lovely and very caring nurse-in-training, who was tipped to marry a handsome doctor by everyone in the group because she was so pretty and kind. We used to go out at night in a group that very soon became a gang. Having such a supportive bunch of friends meant that there was always someone to go to when something went wrong on the wards, when Matron told you off or you were simply having a bad day. There was a real sense of all being in this together.

We were taught to care for the patients in a way that I don't think they are cared for today. We had to make sure they were thoroughly washed; we did their teeth and hair. If they weren't eating or drinking, we cleaned their mouth every couple of hours. If they couldn't feed themselves, we fed them. They were made comfortable, nurtured and cared for. I don't think you get that in hospital now, partly because the nurses are too busy; also because there aren't enough of them and they're often preoccupied with paperwork. There's a lot of technology now as well, which there wasn't in those days.

There seemed to be much more respect for the patient then. Nobody was called by their first name and I think that was a good thing, because if you're doing something intimate to somebody, it's not really appropriate to be calling them 'Bobby' or 'Sarah'. 'Mrs So-and-so' or 'Sir' is much more polite and it's important to be respectful when you're doing such personal things.

So much was different. The matron used to come round every day and talk to every single patient to make sure they were all right. It was also very much stricter then: if a nurse was found sitting on a bed chatting to a patient, she was in big trouble. You weren't even allowed to touch the bed. You could stand beside the patient and talk to them, but sitting down on the bed was forbidden and there was no bending the rules.

The student nurses did all the cleaning. We were the lowest of the low! We used to scrub out the lockers every day and assiduously change the beds. The beds were also scrubbed and thoroughly disinfected between patients, which doesn't always happen now. So there was a lot of cleaning, and although it was tough going on the student nurses, it definitely paid off. Matron policed everybody fiercely, which meant that nothing was overlooked.

After a few months, just as I was beginning to find my feet and gain confidence on the wards, a bombshell dropped – and it was to change my life forever. I had been feeling nauseous for several weeks, which wasn't at all like me. I was a fit and healthy eighteen-year-old and I was totally puzzled. It seems hopelessly naive now when I look back, especially considering I was a nursing student, but things were just so different then. After weeks of wondering what on earth could be wrong with me, I had to face the fact that not only was I exhausted and nauseous all the time, but my period was now long overdue. I was pregnant.

2

Motherhood

At first I didn't know where to turn. I knew my parents would be horrified by my news and I dreaded having to tell them. My mother had never spoken to me about anything connected with reproduction. She was a woman who couldn't even use the word 'pregnant'. I had absorbed some basic information somewhere along the line, and a very strong sense that sex was not something that nice girls should even be thinking about before they were married. I was hopelessly ignorant. That was of course totally normal at the time. Contraceptives were not as readily available as they are to young people today and the Pill had not been on the market very long, so it was quite common for unmarried girls to get pregnant, but it was hugely frowned upon. It is hard to imagine it now, but at that time single pregnant girls had few options. If they wanted to keep their child they had to get married – and even this option carried a stigma with it, as a 'shotgun wedding' still brought shame on a family.

Abortions were hard to arrange, and were frowned on much more than they are today. There were no benefits for single mothers as there are now and therefore a lot of babies were adopted. This was obviously good news for infertile couples, but a desperately sad outcome for many pregnant girls.

My mind whirred, trying to take in the enormity of what was happening. I felt even sicker than before at the thought of all the people I had to tell and how they would react. I knew there was a firestorm of anger and disappointment approaching, but I couldn't avoid it, because I desperately wanted to keep my baby. I was terrified about how my boyfriend would take the news, even though I knew he loved me, because marriage was something that was still on the distant horizon for us. I decided to confide in my fellow students first, knowing that they wouldn't be shocked or judge me. So one evening in the nurses' residence, I plucked up courage and revealed my plight to a couple of the girls I felt closest to. Needless to say, they were full of kind words and sympathy. Then Debbie confessed that she had given a baby up for adoption the previous year. She begged me not to do the same as it had broken her heart. 'Don't give your baby away,' she said tearfully. 'I regret it so much.'

Thankfully my boyfriend, John, didn't have to think twice when I told him the news – straight away he suggested that we get married. That was a huge relief and I started to feel a tiny spark of joy about becoming a mother flickering among all the worry and heartache. I was devastated to give up the career I had waited so long to pursue, but I could not have parted with my baby.

At that point, I was about three months pregnant, which meant that I must have conceived around the start of my training. I don't know why it happened then, but I suspect that the devastating loss of my grandmother may have had something to do with the timing. When one soul goes, another arrives, they say . . . That thought was strangely comforting.

Before I left, I was summoned to an interview with Matron. This was a terrifying prospect, because we were all scared stiff of her. She was a truly formidable figure. When I told her I was pregnant and leaving, I was shaking in my boots. Her reaction was very severe. She said I'd let myself down, I'd let her down, I'd let the hospital down and I'd let my family down. 'Do you think it's right to sleep with somebody before you're married?' she asked me sternly.

'No,' I mumbled, feeling thoroughly ashamed of myself. Although John was my first and only boyfriend, I didn't really think it was right that I had slept with him, because my upbringing had been very Victorian and it had been drummed into us that sex was taboo. I had justified it to myself because we were planning to be together forever, but Matron obviously didn't agree that this was a good enough reason to compromise my virtue. The moral climate was totally different in those days: God forbid that you even contemplated having sex before you made it down the aisle!

Matron told me that she could arrange a termination in the private ward if I wished, and there would be no more said about it. I declined her offer on the spot. It was unthinkable to me. She probably thought she was making me a very reasonable proposal, but it struck me as a horrific idea. 'I'm not doing that!' I thought. I'm not against people having terminations, but I don't think I could have done it.

Even more terrifying than telling John, or telling Matron, was telling my parents that I was pregnant. I had been putting it off for as long as possible, and I felt just as terrible as I'd expected to when I finally found the courage to tell them. They had been so proud of me when I started my training that it felt awful to be letting them down so badly. It also weighed heavily on me that my grandmother had wanted to be a nurse, but her family could not afford to pay for the training. Now I had let my chance go and I only had myself to blame.

My mother was disappointed and cross. 'Well, you've ruined your life, haven't you?' she said. She really wanted me to finish my nursing training and have a career. Still, that didn't mean she wasn't going to be supportive of my decision. There was no way she was going to turn her back on me. It was a different story with my father, who couldn't contain his anger and told me to have a termination or leave home. 'All that money we spent on your private education and this is what you do!' he railed.

Added to the matron's lecture and my inbuilt guilt and shame, this reaction completely squashed that spark of joy I had felt at the prospect of being a mother. When John had reacted so positively, I had dared to hope that the other people in my life would too. Still, I wasn't alone and I knew it. There were millions of women who had it worse than I did, who were abandoned by their baby's father and totally cast off by their family. Some of the more vulnerable ones were even put in psychiatric hospital for being pregnant 'out of wedlock', as it was termed in the 1960s. So I got off lightly, really.

I was sad to leave my new friends and even though we kept in touch for a while we ended up drifting apart. It was inevitable, really. We hadn't known each other long enough to forge lifelong friendships and we all went in different directions.

All except Barbara, that is. Lovely Barbara stayed in touch and, true to our predictions, went on to marry a medical student when she finished her training. She and her husband lived in hospital accommodation and it wasn't long before she became pregnant. But then one morning, a few months into the pregnancy, her husband woke up and found her dead in bed. There was a rare complication in her pregnancy that went undetected and could not have been prevented.

It was shattering to hear the news, and truly one of those moments in life when you realise the extent of your blessings. Although we'd kept in touch, the last time I had seen Barbara was when I was leaving training school, more or less in disgrace. Beautiful Barbara was sweet to me as I said my goodbyes, and I felt a pang of envy as I contemplated the life that she would now have, and I would not. When Barbara died, I felt so awful when I remembered the envy I had felt. It struck me that Barbara had done everything the right way, just how I would have liked to have done it: she finished her training and met a lovely doctor, they got married and they were having a baby. She had everything to live for – and yet look how she ended up.

Even more tragically, her husband was so distraught by her death that a short time later he took his own life. Going up to London for their memorial service was really upsetting. A picture of a clown with tears was hung on the wall at the hospital to honour them. Three of them lost – what a tragedy for their families.

No longer welcome at home by my father, I moved in with John's mother. She had been in my situation herself in 1948, so she was anxious to help us. Her ill-fated marriage had ended after a short time, so John had never known his father well, and she never married again. John's new role would be unfamiliar territory for him.

We had a lovely wedding, which my mother attended but my father did not. My mother had continued to give me her love and support, popping round to see me at John's mum's, really keen not to miss out on my pregnancy and so excited at the prospect of becoming a grandmother. But I never saw my father. I didn't hold it against him, as I could understand why he'd reacted the way he did. I suppose in some ways I thought he was justified. It had been so drummed into me that I was to have a career, and 'keep out of trouble'. I simply couldn't shake the guilt I felt about letting him down.

After a little while, John and I were lucky enough to find a little flat to rent in a town nearby, where we prepared for the arrival of our baby. That joy I had felt was growing stronger and stronger, despite my father's continuing refusal to see me and my own lingering guilt. I knew that I really loved this baby already, and couldn't wait to meet him or her. I had always wanted to be a mother. It had happened sooner than I would have wanted, but John and I were in love and committed to making things work. I got a temporary clerical job so that I could set aside some money for the baby's arrival; despite my inability to type, my college training came in useful around the office – my mother was right in the end!

I attended the local hospital antenatal classes but found them unhelpful and embarrassing, partly because I still felt guilty about my circumstances. I was not yet nineteen and looked very young, so I imagine everyone guessed that my baby wasn't exactly planned.

Despite my excitement about impending motherhood, I was also anxious and scared throughout the pregnancy. The problem was that nobody could reassure you in those days that everything was going to be all right with the baby. My big fear was that I might be punished for having sex outside marriage by being given a baby that wasn't quite 'right'. There was no way of knowing if your child was healthy, because there was no scanning technology. You just had to get on with it. Still, I put my apprehensions to the back of my mind and said to myself, 'I'll love the baby whatever, because it's ours.'

Apart from the antenatal classes, I really didn't have much contact at all with the medical professionals. I didn't see a community midwife; I didn't even have a GP in the area, because I'd just moved there and my doctor was still in the next town. I was so stupid! I didn't think to ask about my options: I saw the midwives at the hospital, but the possibility of having a home birth was never even mentioned and I just went along with the system. You probably had to be very settled and living in a nice house for them to approve a home birth, whereas we were living in a flat at the top of a building. You'd think I would have been a bit more on the ball after doing a bit of nursing, but in those days pregnancy and childbirth were barely talked about. I didn't have any friends who had babies and my mum certainly wouldn't discuss anything with me – she was still a bit embarrassed about the whole situation, and was never able to talk about personal matters with me.

Back then, antenatal classes were just for women, so John wasn't able to attend. It was probably just as well, because they told you outright lies about giving birth, assuring you that it wouldn't hurt. It was just a load of rubbish. Since I had very little idea of what giving birth involved, I remained totally clueless. It may seem as if I was very naive, but nobody talked about bodily parts and bodily functions back then and birth wasn't a regular feature of TV dramas, as it is now. The whole idea of it mortified me. At one point, we sat on the floor, rather pointlessly pretending to have contractions, and I remember that I was too embarrassed to sit with my knees apart, because I'd been brought up *never* to sit with my knees apart. 'If you don't open your legs, that baby's never going to come out!' the midwife chided. I blushed awkwardly. I felt so uncomfortable with it all.

She told us to tap out a tune with our fingers during our contractions, the idea being that humming and tapping would take your mind off the pain. Distraction technique, I think they call it now. Even though I had no idea what she was talking about, I chose 'Ob-la-di, Ob-la-da' as my tune, which was one of the Beatles' hits at the time. I dutifully tapped it out at every antenatal class I attended, hoping the Fab Four would help ease my baby into the world.

But when the birth day finally arrived, nothing happened the way I had been told it would. It's true that nothing can fully prepare you for the reality of childbirth, but it's safe to say that the little I'd been told was completely useless to me. I had a really quick labour. It only lasted three and a half hours and was very intense, right from the start. There was no slow build-up in which I could get used to the contractions. It wasn't like that at all. I woke up at home and bang, I was in severe pain. So there was no 'Ob-la-di, Ob-la-da'! Everything I had been taught went out of the window and instead of humming and tapping, I was screaming in agony.

I'd been told that each contraction would rise to a peak and die away, but there was no let up. I didn't know it at the time, but this was because I had what's known as a 'back-ache' or posterior labour, where the baby is pressing against your spine. It's incredibly tough on your back and the pain is there all the time; nothing I did made it any better. Now I know that there are strategies like back-rubbing that can help, but I didn't know any of that at the time.

The pain was so bad that I honestly thought I was dying; I remember lying on the bed screaming my head off, to the extent that the people next door said they thought there was a murder being committed in our flat! I was completely hysterical and out of control. My mind was overwhelmed with sheer terror; I was frightened out of my wits.

My husband had no idea what to do. Why would he? He telephoned the hospital twice for advice. 'It's too early to come in with a first baby,' the midwife told him sharply. 'She'll be ages yet.'

'Can't you hear her screaming in the background?' he asked frantically, but his fears were dismissed as those of an anxious first-time father.

Eventually, when I started making pushing noises, he called an ambulance. I didn't actually want to go to hospital, because I dreaded coming up against the disapproval of the medical staff and I was worried I'd be made to feel like a naughty girl for 'getting into trouble'. I didn't want to experience the embarrassment that I'd felt at my antenatal classes, where the women seemed so much older and more settled than I was. But in the circumstances, we didn't know what else to do. Whatever the midwife at the hospital thought, it seemed as if the baby was definitely on its way.

When the two ambulance men arrived, much to my indignation, they peered under the blanket which was covering me. 'How dare you?' I thought, my modesty overruling my fear for a few short seconds.

'It looks like we need to call for a midwife urgently!' one of them exclaimed. I've no idea what he saw to elicit this reaction, but it was probably blood. I think I was actually pushing too, but since I was screaming in pain and fear, I couldn't talk coherently or explain what I was feeling. Poor John was scared out of his wits as well, understandably.

I don't know how long it was before the midwife appeared at our flat, but I do remember that she came on her pushbike. That's how it was in 1969. Everything changed with her arrival; she was young and blonde and she had the situation under control within minutes.

'Now Agnes, that's enough of that noise,' were her first words to me, once she had asked John what my name was. 'Come on, let's have this baby!' she added firmly but kindly. She was fantastic.

'Thank God someone's here to help me!' I thought and I shut up straight away.

'It's going to be all right. The baby will be here soon,' she soothed. 'There's nothing wrong. Everything's normal.'

She coaxed me and reassured me and told me what to do; my panic and fear subsided in the face of her quiet confidence. I became calm in the knowledge that she was in charge. I still remember the sheer terror very vividly, although of course the pain is a distant memory. But the agony of being so scared that I thought I would die has never left me. Then this saviour arrived and, as if she had flicked a switch, everything was better. The pain was still there, of course, but the despair that comes from pure terror had gone. It was an important turning-point for me in more ways than one, because in that moment I knew that I was not going to die and began to relax into the birth. Everything became easier as a result. And I'm sure it also had a lot to do with my subsequent decision to try again to become a midwife. In fact, everything that happened after the midwife arrived contributed to the feeling that one day perhaps I could be on the other side, helping women give birth and learn to look after their babies.

The midwife had put me on one side and she was telling me exactly what to do. I felt a calmness and concentration come over me, as if somehow I knew exactly what my body was capable of, and could trust it. I was focused purely on the goal of bringing our child into the world. Matthew was born shortly afterwards. The midwife eased him out and in that instant I felt a rush of joy and exhilaration and pure unbounded love. I was crying, John was teary and Matthew was bawling as the midwife washed him and handed him to me.

In the end, despite the awful unexpected pain and the rush and the horror of thinking I was going to die, my baby was here and he was beautiful. I felt very empowered and very pleased with myself, especially as I hadn't needed to go to hospital. I was like everybody is just after they've given birth: during labour they're screaming, swearing and trying to bite you – and then as soon as the baby's out, they change completely. 'Isn't the baby lovely? I'm so happy!' they declare. I was just the same. I thought I was so clever – the bee's knees!

Of course, it wasn't long before I was reminded of my ignorance again. When the midwife left, she said, 'Just wee in a bucket next to the bed; don't get up to go to the toilet.' I did as directed, but was shocked to see a mass of blood in the bottom of the bucket. I didn't know that blood came out of you after having a baby! Nobody had told me to expect it. That's how uninformed I was.

In a panic, I made my husband phone the midwife. 'Tell her that I'm haemorrhaging to death and she's got to come back!'

She returned on her bike and took a look in the bucket. 'What's the matter with you? That's normal!' she said, and off she cycled again. She must have thought I was really stupid, but if you've never experienced really heavy periods and you suddenly see a huge flow of blood and clots coming out of you, it can be quite frightening. You could quite easily think that you were bleeding to death. So I always warn women who have just given birth about this, just in case they don't know to expect it, because it really is quite scary.

I hadn't realised at the time – my mind was on more important matters – but the ambulance men were still there through all of this. They stayed until after the birth was over.

Finally, they came to say goodbye. I couldn't even look at them; I was so embarrassed. 'Thanks for letting us watch the birth,' the older one said. 'My mate's never seen a baby being born before, so he was quite pleased.'

I was mortified. I was so shy that I couldn't even take my clothes off in front of my husband, so the fact that they had seen all of this appalled me. These days anything goes, and I think most people would just be glad that they were there helping, but to have strange men watching me then, oh dear!

I couldn't really care too much about it though. I was in a little love bubble with my precious new baby. I adored Matthew from the very first moment I laid eyes on him, and although life with a newborn baby is a rude shock to the system for everyone, I was utterly happy. I loved all the attention and praise that came in the days to follow and soon the trauma was completely forgotten. When my student nurse friends came to visit I felt a pang of regret at my lost chances, but I hoped I would still become a nurse one day and I adored having a baby to look after. I loved it all so much that I was pregnant again after three months . . . deliberately this time!

The only sadness in my life was the rift with my father, whom I hadn't seen for six months. So I was really pleased to receive a letter from him, not long after Matthew was born.

'There is too much unhappiness in the world without me adding to it, so please come to lunch on Sunday,' he implored.

I was over the moon to be taken back into the family again and it was a relief for my mum, who had suffered agonies during the time when my father and I weren't speaking. I wondered whether she had been working on my behalf, trying to talk him round. I had begun to lose hope that we would ever be reconciled, because my dad was very stubborn, but he just couldn't bear not to be a part of his grandson's life. He loved Matthew, as he did all the rest of his grandchildren when they came along. Perhaps it had also occurred to him that as he wasn't perfect, he shouldn't expect perfection in his children. His alcoholism had blighted our family life from my early childhood, and I think his change of heart about me was an acknowledgement, however oblique, of the pain his illness had inflicted on everyone. Whatever the reasons, I was just overjoyed that we were in contact and that I was back in the bosom of the family.

John, Matthew and I soon moved to a nice little house in a quiet and friendly Kent village and our second son Edward was born at home. This time I was registered with a local GP and he was very supportive. In fact, he suggested a home birth to me, saying I'd be a drain on the health service if I went into hospital. 'We haven't got the money to deal with healthy young people like you!' he said.

Everything was planned, so it was a whole different ball game. I had felt so empowered after my first childbirth that I had no hesitation in taking the doctor's suggestion seriously and opting for a home birth, and I enjoyed my pregnancy hugely. I was less anxious this time around and no longer felt guilty about being an only-just-married mother. On top of that, I was reconciled with my father and I couldn't have felt more positive. I already knew the community midwife who would be coming to the birth, because she'd seen me at every appointment. I trusted her and knew she would look after me. What a difference that made to the pregnancy and birth!

My husband rang her soon after my contractions started. 'Have I got time to have my breakfast?' she asked him.

'Has she got time to have her breakfast?' he asked me.

'No!' I yelled. 'Tell her to come now!'

The birth was a piece of cake, because I knew what to expect. Again, it was really quick – two hours from start to finish – and very intense, but I wasn't scared because I knew why everything was happening. This is just me, I realised. I have very fast labours. It's not always a good thing when it's quick, because the intensity means it's very painful, but I knew there would be an end to it. Everything felt very much under control. The midwife arrived with a student midwife; Edward was born and that was that. All was calm and there was no screaming at all, not even from the toddler! It was lovely; just how it should have been.

I could see a massive difference between my second birth and the first. Physically, it had been more or less the same, because it was really quick, but I'd had so much more support this time. This is how a birth should be, I thought. Of course, it was also different because I was a mother already. Becoming a mother is such a huge thing. Suddenly you're responsible for this tiny person and you never know how you're going to deal with it. But the second time around you're a mother already, so you haven't got that part of it to adapt to. I always say to people that the second pregnancy is the nicest, because you don't have all the horror of thinking, 'Oh my God, what's going to happen?' You know what's going to happen, you know how to deal with it and you get another baby to look after, so it's really lovely.

The next eighteen months were very contented ones, or so I thought at the time. When I look back I suppose I can see that things were sometimes strained between John and me, partly because being married wasn't really how I'd expected it to be. You couldn't really be selfish anymore and I liked to get my own way all the time! And of course fathers didn't get involved so much with their children then, so John was out to work every day and then came home and saw the children for a little while before I put supper on the table. That's how it was supposed to be.

Still, as far as I was concerned I was very happily married, so it came as a terrible shock when John announced out of the blue that he had met someone else. He worked with her; there were just the two of them at work all day, five days a week, so it was an accident waiting to happen really. I felt so stupid – the wife sitting at home with the kids who hadn't seen any of this coming. It was humiliating, and after the euphoria of parenthood it was a brutal reminder that happy-ever-after is far more common in fairy tales than in real life. I felt terribly low for weeks, and it was a huge effort to drag myself around and keep everything running as normal for the kids.

There are two sides to every story and I'm sure I wasn't always easy to live with, so I don't blame John completely. I think we were both too young for the situation in which we found ourselves and neither of us knew how to adapt to married life. There was also a real lack of communication between us; we just didn't know how to talk to each other.

The upshot was that we parted amid a lot of tears and recriminations, although things eventually settled down after he left. I waited for my parents to say, 'We told you so!' But they didn't. They were completely supportive. Still, I felt I'd let them down again and disappointed them. 'I'm getting my just desserts now,' I thought. 'Here I am, twenty-three years old with two children, on my own.'

These days you can choose to be a single mum and it doesn't matter a jot, but in the early seventies it was something to be ashamed of. It was a lonely and often sad time for me, but I managed to get through it. Having to look after the children helped me enormously. Small children are entertaining and endlessly affectionate as well as hard work, and they were a joy to me when everything else felt like the life had gone out of it. But they were demanding, and I had virtually no independent identity. After a while, I decided I had to get a job, not only to earn money for us, but also to save my sanity. My parents helped me out a lot but I didn't want to rely on them all the time; I had to stand on my own two feet.

For a while I worked in a nightclub in the nearby town. I loved it, as the staff were very kind to me when they found out I was a single mother. It was also a fun place to work and I made some good friends. I had a wonderful neighbour, Rosemary, who was a single mum herself, and she looked after the boys for me when I was at work. It worked out well all round; the arrangement gave me peace of mind and gave her some much-needed extra money.

All the female staff at the nightclub wore orange hot pants and orange and black patterned chiffon blouses. It was 1972 and we thought we looked fashionable and sexy, because hot pants were all the rage. I usually worked in the restaurant section, and often when I entered the kitchen Mrs King, the lady chef, snorted at me, 'Get that big orange bottom out of my way, please!' It was all very good-natured, as she was quite large herself!

Despite my intrusions into her cooking area, Mrs King

always gave me a large steak to take home, as there was no time to eat during the evening. The manager ordered the meat supplies and he used to receive a joint of meat from the butcher as a thankyou for the order. Since he lived in digs and had no need for the extra food, he used to give it to me. The children and I had never been so well fed!

We were a close-knit team and we enjoyed our work. At around 2am, when everybody had gone home, we used to sit round and have a drink together. It was good clean fun. It was a great time for me, as it kind of felt as if I were experiencing the life I would have had if I hadn't got married so young. And as far as I was concerned, working in a nightclub was just as entertaining as going to one.

Eventually, after a couple of years, I had to leave because life was about to change again. John had split up from his partner and suggested we get back together. We moved to a new house back in our home town, but my happiness was only to last six months. When John's ex-partner heard that we had got back together, she threatened to kill herself and so he left me and went back to her. This time I was even more distraught than I had been the first time he left and I became more and more depressed.

It was a desperate time. I felt like a total failure. I had been abandoned by the father of my children, not once, but twice. I didn't think I would ever have another relationship; I couldn't even imagine wanting to have one. I loved my children but I could barely function enough to keep us all going. Fortunately, I had endless support from my parents, who lived five minutes away and who, to their credit, never said that our marriage had been a mistake.

It took me months to begin to recover my sense of purpose and any optimism about the future. Once again, it was my children who pulled me though. My children and the thought, lurking somewhere in the back of my mind ever since that moment when the midwife had saved me from the terror of my first childbirth, that what I really wanted to do was train to be a midwife.

That thought got stronger and clearer until it became a definite goal. When I was ready to get a job again, I decided to work as a nursing auxiliary at the local general hospital. As my children were five and six years old, I had to be able to fit work around their needs, so I couldn't contemplate nurse training yet. But I was certain about where I wanted to end up. I didn't want to be a nobody forever. It might take a while, but I was determined to do something with my life.

I absolutely loved the work in the hospital. I had a bit more life experience now and found it easier to communicate with the patients. There were some lovely nurses too; they never once treated me as if I was beneath them and sometimes they let me carry out procedures which were probably not in my remit as an untrained assistant.

One day a friendly nurse who knew about my career ambitions was waiting for me when I arrived on the ward. 'I've just found out there's a two-year midwifery training course for people who aren't qualified nurses already,' she said excitedly. 'It's based at a hospital about fifteen miles away. You should definitely apply for it.'

I couldn't wait to telephone them and find out about the course. I had always thought that I would have to do three years' general training before I could do the one-year midwifery training. Here was the fast-track and it seemed perfect for me. When I enquired, it seemed I had enough qualifications, but the course was full. I begged them to take my details in case anyone dropped out. As luck would have it, the course secretary phoned back two days later to offer me a place. I was over the moon. Finally, after so many years of struggle and heartache, I was getting a bit of a break.

At this point I had not thought about childcare, transport, shift work and any of the other obstacles, but now I had to start planning. I've always found that if you're determined, you'll find a way to do it. My family rallied round and after initially questioning whether it was feasible, they were really supportive. My sister, herself a single mother, moved in. She also worked, so we helped each other out with the kids, and I took in a lodger to boost our income. My mother didn't have a job outside the home so she was happy to care for her grandchildren. It always gave her enormous pleasure. I would never have wanted to leave my children with childminders and I couldn't afford to anyway, not on a student's salary. My father helped me to buy a car which, although old, was trustworthy. Despite his drinking problem, my father still managed to run his flooring business successfully. He was never good at showing emotion but he always helped me financially.

It had taken until I was twenty-seven, but I was now on the road to a career again and my self-esteem soared.

3

Back to School
1976

I was very excited on my first day of training and so proud to be called a pupil midwife. We didn't get straight into learning the art and science of midwifery; that was to come later. The first eight weeks of the course were spent with a group of new students who were learning to be general nurses. This was to give us a thorough grounding in how the human body functions and how to care for people in hospital. As I had already done this introductory training when I was eighteen – and also worked as an auxiliary nurse – I didn't find it daunting at all. In fact, I loved every minute of it.

Of course not all pregnancies are straightforward and not all women are healthy, and therefore it is necessary to know about the body in sickness and in health. After the introductory course the pupil midwives were to spend six months working as student nurses in the general hospital. We were placed on wards where we could gain experience in medicine, surgery, gynaecology and theatre techniques.

In the years since I had initially trained as a nurse, the uniform had gone through a transformation. Now we had a plain white dress to wear; not a good colour when working near blood! And it was made from polyester with cotton, which made it a bit hot and uncomfortable. We wore different coloured belts to denote our status, from first-year trainee to midwifery sister, but of course we all looked alike to the patients, who generally had no idea who was senior to whom. We didn't wear hats at all, which I was slightly disappointed about, because I had a soft spot for the meringues from my earlier training days, even though they were difficult to construct. Still, I was relieved that tights had become popular, which meant we didn't have to put up with the discomfort or inconvenience of stockings and suspenders.

In the mixed wards the male patients found it very amusing to be cared for by a midwife in training rather than a general nursing student. The ward joker (and there always is one!) would shout out whenever he spotted one of us arriving on duty, 'Quick, Nurse, the baby's coming!'

This always amused his fellow patients and their visitors. Sometimes we would retaliate by marching up to the joker's bed with a stern expression and the appearance of real intent.

'Right, dear, let's get these pyjama trousers off so the baby doesn't get tangled up in them!'

Funnily enough, the joker never wanted to comply with this request and suddenly decided the baby wasn't coming after all . . . it had been a false alarm. Of course the feared and respected ward sister was never around when this banter was taking place, as it is very unlikely she would have been amused.

I really enjoyed this period of my training. I quickly regained my confidence on the wards and began to forge good friendships with some of my colleagues. Those early days were also marked by a couple of very sad incidents though. One day, which happened to be my birthday, a thirty-year-old man was admitted to the ward with a suspected heart attack. Walking past his bed, I glanced at his heart monitor and, although not really understanding the technology, I noticed it had rather a strange pattern on it. I went to tell the ward sister, but she dismissed me abruptly with a look of annoyance. 'What do you know about heart patients? You're a pupil midwife!' she sneered.

It was very hierarchical in the NHS in those days. Everybody lived in fear of the sister and you didn't actually speak to her unless you had a good reason. The staff nurse was on the level beneath her and the students were below everyone. Nobody talked to us at all, so for a student midwife to speak up was outrageous. But I've never been able to keep my head down, which has probably got me into trouble a lot more than I'd like. I always speak up when I think there's a need to. I just can't stop myself.

As it turned out, it probably wouldn't have made a scrap of difference if the ward sister had gone to check the heart monitor. A short while later, the poor man had a second massive heart attack and died. I was shocked and upset, as I always was when I was witness to a death. I never got used to it.

I remember being particularly moved by the case of a young woman patient who had a devoted husband and a small baby. She was taken to the operating theatre for an investigation into the cause of severe abdominal pain. Sadly, when the surgeon opened her abdomen he discovered she had inoperable liver cancer; her husband was told she only had a short time to live. I felt so sorry for him sitting by her bed cuddling their baby while he waited for her to wake up properly after the anaesthetic. I wondered what he was going to tell her. I felt powerless to help him. These heartbreaking moments become almost a matter of routine when you work in a hospital, but of course every single one is a personal tragedy for those involved and unbelievably painful to witness.

One patient, a very charming lady who was the mother of four adult sons and a daughter, started talking to me in earnest about her prognosis. Patients always seem to ask the most junior staff the most serious questions.

'Nurse, am I going to die?' she asked softly.

I knew she had terminal cancer, but her children did not want her to know, so obviously I was not allowed to confirm what I am sure she suspected. This was back in the days when it was standard practice to withhold information from the patient if that was what their relatives wished, a state of affairs that fortunately would never happen now. Luckily I remembered something our tutor had said when we discussed what we would do in this situation.

'There is one sure thing in life, and that is that we are all going to die sometime,' I replied simply. I'm glad to say that she seemed satisfied with my answer.

Often the patients were much easier to deal with than our senior colleagues. On my first day on duty on the surgical wards, I wandered into the sitting room attached to the theatre area when it was time for my tea break. There I joined a few members of staff who were enjoying a brief respite from their duties. The sister in charge looked up at me in horror.

'You should not be in here, Nurse! Get out!' she squawked. I looked at her in surprise. 'Students take their tea in the kitchen,' she added haughtily.

Well, the kitchen was a very small, airless room with no comfortable chairs. I felt so humiliated in front of all the other staff. 'I'm a twenty-seven-year-old mother,' I thought. 'How can she speak to me like that?' But it didn't matter what age you were or what experience you'd had in life; there was no choice but to conform. Still, I vowed then that I would never treat students badly once I was qualified. And I never have.

Another time, a sister in charge told me to go and put another bag of fluid into a patient's drip. 'Are you sure? She's already had two,' I said.

'Just do it. Don't question me!' she snapped.

So I did what she said. The patient then experienced an overload of fluid and ended up having a fit. It wasn't my fault, because I was only a student; it was the sister who took the rap for it. Of course, she never referred to the incident afterwards.

I came up against situations like that throughout my training. You weren't supposed to speak out of turn or make suggestions, but I found it very difficult not to. My colleagues called me a rebel. 'Stop getting yourself into trouble! Keep your mouth shut,' they advised. But I don't think I was a rebel. It's just that I don't like bad practice or injustice and I will always speak up if I think someone's health or wellbeing is being jeopardised. If I see something that needs pointing out, I'll speak up.

Power goes to people's heads, but by no means everyone was affected, thankfully. One day, I was actually invited by one of the surgeons to stand next to him and watch the contents of someone's abdomen being pulled out! It was a nerve-racking experience, but absolutely fascinating. He described everything he was doing – and taught me so much about the inner workings of the human body in the process that I had no time to feel squeamish. I was surprised and grateful that this doctor was so kind to me, as I was used to being treated like something stuck on the bottom of a shoe.

I was always very grateful of any opportunity to stand and watch in the operating theatre, but I wasn't very happy with the uniform. We wore tight-fitting turbans made from a J-cloth-type material which, combined with green theatre pyjamas, made it impossible to look glamorous enough to attract a sexy anaesthetist!

The gynaecology ward was probably the place I gained the most useful and relevant knowledge in my first six months of training. It was often quite an emotional place to work, because there were women on the ward who were suffering from miscarriages as well as women who were going to have terminations. There were women recovering from hysterectomies, who saw the operation as the end of their fertile years, and women having surgery to investigate their lack of fertility. Each patient needed nursing, as well as individual emotional, moral or spiritual support during her particular ordeal. There was a lot of sadness and tears and I felt upset that I had neither the knowledge nor experience to help properly. It was so humbling to realise how much I had to learn, not about the anatomy or the procedures, but about how best to alleviate the complex individual pain each patient was living through.

For a long time I thought that if you had a miscarriage, well, it was sad, but you could always try again. I didn't understand how it felt until I'd spoken to some of the women on the gynaecology ward. Then I began to realise that it was a much bigger trauma than I'd imagined and that it didn't matter at what stage you lost a baby, because it always represented the loss of a child's future.

Certainly, a lot of the nurses didn't seem to think it was a big deal. I remember taking my sister-in-law into hospital when she was having a miscarriage, after I qualified, and it was more like she'd lost a shoe than a baby. There was no sympathy whatsoever. It was awful. That's when I started to see the difference between the nurses and the midwives, I think. Midwives do a lot more training in the psychology of childbearing, which is perhaps why some nurses don't have much sympathy when it comes to miscarriages.

I also learnt that having a hysterectomy has quite a profound psychological impact on a lot of women, even if they've already had their children, because they equate the end of their reproductive years and the removal of their womb with a loss of femininity. Terminations can also be very upsetting and some people don't realise that they're going to be so affected by the procedure until it actually happens. Interestingly, a lot of women consciously and deliberately get pregnant soon after a termination.

I found I was too inexperienced in life to understand the different emotions around termination, miscarriage and hysterectomy, but I did my best. I learnt a lot from the women when they opened up about how they felt; as well as physically looking after people, our job was to offer a sympathetic ear. Many of the women seemed to want to talk to anyone who would listen. They'd be pouring their hearts out while you were making the bed and bringing them a cup of tea. I absorbed everything I heard and stored it all up for future reference. And I never forgot that my first job was to comfort my patients.

Finally the day came when I was back on the maternity wing for good. Here was where we would learn all about the physiology of childbearing and the art and science of midwifery. I had to learn about the emotional and spiritual aspects for myself, as that was not part of the curriculum. This was the mid-seventies. Women's liberation was only just beginning to make a difference to the way we did things, and although it seems incredible today, women's feelings were rarely taken into account. They were not routinely consulted and their wishes were certainly not deferred to except by a very few enlightened individuals. There was an unspoken rule that the medical professionals knew best. Their advice was usually taken without question.

I thought it was wrong that the women didn't get a say in anything at all. They were never asked if they agreed to things; they were just told what to do and they got on with it. Some colleagues have since confided to me that they preferred the way things were, back when the women didn't know anything and were more compliant. It's true that they didn't complain and just let things happen to them, but I don't think that's how it should be.

I respected the doctors very much, because they had so much experience, but they weren't always right, and no-one really seemed to care about how the women felt. The emotional and spiritual aspects of having a baby were being ignored and I didn't agree with that.

Three bureaucratic, ageing spinsters called nursing officers ran the maternity department. They had probably trained at the time when married women were not accepted into the nursing profession. They may even have lost beloved fiancés during the war years. Unmarried and without children, they had dedicated their lives to their careers. They were quite fierce and only showed kindness to the mothers and their babies. They had no time for fathers, doctors or students, all of whom they believed should be seen and not heard! This was in the days when men were still supposed to be pacing the corridors and keeping out of the way.

I felt fathers should be more involved in the whole process, especially the delivery. My husband had been, and it didn't kill him. John saw our two babies being born; no-one told him to leave the room and he didn't think he should, either! He found it an emotional experience to hold each baby immediately after birth. Some fathers find birth a bit disgusting, but John certainly never voiced any such opinions to me, and it didn't affect our relationship that he saw me give birth, although I think it can disturb some men.

Of course, it didn't matter what I thought about fathers being included – rules and regulations abounded and they were not to be questioned. Sometimes the antenatal clinic seemed to be like a production line, with women passing through like robots. And just as I used to be sent to the headmistress at school for a dressing-down, so I was sent to my tutor, on one occasion, for being too familiar with the patients in the clinic. I had simply tried to treat them as individuals and show them some respect, but my efforts earned me a reprimand from the clinic sister.

'There is no time for idle chat, Nurse. A great number of women have to be shepherded through very quickly and seen by the doctor.'

Actually, most of them didn't need to see a doctor at all, as they were perfectly healthy and had no complications; a chat with a midwife would probably have been much more useful to them. But in the 1970s, doctors still did a lot of unnecessary consultations.

I tried to argue with her. 'I only treat the patients as I wish to be treated myself,' I said in my defence. 'I've been pregnant and I know what it feels like to be scared and anxious and needing reassurance from someone friendly.'

However, my tutor was a childless spinster who didn't understand my point of view, so I might as well have been talking to a brick wall. Unfortunately, after that my card was marked.

And it wasn't only the senior staff I had problems with.

The gory aspects of the job also took a bit of getting used to. For instance, taking blood from women in the antenatal clinic was a bit of an ordeal for me too. I was often to be found with my head between my knees, feeling worse than my victim! After a particularly difficult attempt, the clinic sister informed me that I was trying to take blood from a tendon instead of a vein. I've always found it surprising that drug addicts find their veins so easily.

Despite such difficulties, I really enjoyed my time in the antenatal clinic. I have always believed it to be an area with a special responsibility. It is usually the first port of call for a pregnant woman coming to hospital and as such it gives a very important first impression. If a woman is treated with kindness and the staff are friendly, it sets the scene for the rest of her pregnancy.

It was the practice at the time to spend some time in every area in the maternity department and because about four thousand babies were born at the hospital in a year, there was plenty of experience to be had in the labour ward. The more modern term for this area is the delivery suite, although personally I have always associated the word 'suite' with a very large room in a posh hotel, where you'd go for a love tryst with someone who may or may not be your partner! Nothing remotely similar takes place in the delivery suite, except that a woman's intimate body parts may be observed and touched from time to time. To me, labour ward seems a much more appropriate name, as we all know that giving birth is extremely hard labour.

As a pupil midwife, I was required to see twenty births before being allowed to deliver a baby myself. Even when I had my 'hands on' for the first few times, a qualified midwife had her hands over mine, because she might have needed to take over if I suddenly started hyperventilating, something that was quite likely if I was trying to show the woman how to pant. Of course, in my case people wondered whether I would actually remain upright long enough to catch the baby! My queasiness had become a bit of a standing joke, but I had got over my worries about it. In actual fact, whenever I really had to toughen up and be responsible for something, I was fine.

Since the midwife had her hands on top of mine, I didn't feel my first delivery was totally mine. Still, it was just so wonderful to think that I helped get this baby out into the world. It was also reassuring to have the midwife there; I couldn't have done anything wrong because she would have kicked me out of the way immediately! I was so nervous that I probably didn't do anything much. She was giving me instructions and I was just following them dumbly.

The mother was quite young and it was her first baby. I don't think she knew or cared that it was my first delivery. I certainly didn't make a point of saying that it was the first time I'd caught a baby; we just marched in there and got on with it, because that's what you did in those days. In fact, I wouldn't have dreamt of telling her I hadn't done it before, whereas I think it would be difficult not to say it today. Women are much more clued up and more likely to say that they want someone experienced. Yet I didn't mind that there was a student midwife present at my second child Edward's birth, or that she caught the baby with the midwife standing close by. It didn't worry me; I just accepted it.

Catching babies is only a small part of midwifery, but obviously it's a very important part. If you know what you're doing, you can often prevent someone from tearing, which makes a huge difference to their recovery after the birth. Just before the head comes out, you don't want the woman to be pushing hard, because the baby can come out too fast and that might cause her to tear. So you try to watch or have your hand there to feel for when the widest part of the baby's head is coming out. You're not holding it back; you're waiting and feeling the baby coming forwards. What normally happens is that the baby comes forwards and then it recedes a little, until you get to a point when it comes forwards but doesn't recede anymore. That's when you know it's on its way. After the head comes out, you have to feel for the umbilical cord and make sure it's not around the baby's neck. If it is, you have to loop it back over its head. Otherwise, the cord may strangle the baby as it comes out.

Over time, and with experience, a midwife learns what it feels like when the baby is going to come out with the next push. That's when you ask the woman not to push and just to pant, so that there's no great force behind the baby and it comes out very slowly. Sometimes it gets a bit stuck and you have to say, 'Right, give me a little push now.' You're just trying to guide the head out really gently. When the head emerges, the baby turns round to get its shoulders in line. It does that all by itself! When the shoulders hit the pelvic floor, they automatically turn, or they should do. Then you have to guide the shoulders out, one shoulder at a time, because they can cause a tear as well.

If you get it wrong, someone can tear quite badly – some people tear right down to the back passage and that's very serious, because then they might have a sphincter that doesn't work, which means they have no control over their bowels. Sometimes it happens and it's not the midwife's fault, because the woman just can't help pushing, but I do think midwives can make a lot of difference if they're careful. However, different midwives have different ways of catching babies and some don't put their hands on; they just let the woman do it herself while they stand by, watching. But I don't like doing that; I think it's much better to be helping out.

There's a curve in the birth canal, so the baby emerges downwards and then you lift it right up to get the rest of the body out. When I was training, everybody was lying on a bed. They weren't allowed to stand up; they had to be horizontal. Now they can be in any position, so you've got to be able to catch the baby from all angles. If the woman is on all fours, it's a different method again, because you do it the opposite way – instead of down and up, you guide the baby up and down.

You don't turn it upside down and smack its bottom next, like most people think you do. You always see it in the films, but I've never seen it in real life. First, you have to make sure the baby's mouth is clear, so that it can start breathing. Sometimes it takes about a minute before a baby cries and that's an awfully long time to wait. You have to be thinking all the time, 'Is it blue? Is it going to breathe? Is it going to come round, or isn't it?' You're feeling either the heart or the cord to make sure it's pulsating. If it's going really slowly, you should start resuscitating the baby. All of these things are going through your mind when you're a midwife.

You have to give it a score out of ten in your head, rating how well it is overall by taking into account whether it's breathing and moving, its heart rate and whether it cries. An inexperienced student can't do all of that; the only thing they can really do the first time is be there and let the baby slide into their hands, wet, slippery and bloody. That's such a momentous thing that you can't think about anything else when you're new to it. You know you should be doing all sorts of calculations, but you can't. If anything needed doing, you hoped the midwife would do it – and obviously that's exactly what happened.

At that first birth I just stood there with the baby in my arms, overwhelmed. Finally I was doing what I had set out to do all those years ago. I was helping another woman in the way that I had been helped myself. It was truly one of the best moments of my entire life. I had tears in my eyes as I looked over at my more experienced colleague. She smiled back at me and I could tell that though she had probably done this hundreds of times, she was moved as well. The truth is, you never become blasé about catching a baby.

Our hands were together and we got the baby out; that was the extent of my involvement, really. The tears spilled over as we lifted it up. Nowadays the midwife will clamp the cord and cut it, wrap the baby up, make sure it's breathing all right and give it to the mother. But at that time, the policy was to give babies a minute of oxygen as soon as they were born. I have no idea why. We don't do it anymore, but they used to think it was a good thing to do. So instead of giving the baby to the mum, you had to put it in its cot and give it oxygen before she could hold it. This was another practice I didn't agree with. 'What's the point of it?' I thought. 'Why does a newborn need oxygen when it's breathing fine?'

It's funny, they used to do a lot of things that had little or no benefit, and it's only over the years that they've decided they're not necessary anymore. When I started training, we were always told that we should make a cut to the woman's perineum, the area between the vagina and the anus, if it was her first baby. But when this was researched, it was found to be completely pointless. She might tear a little bit, but that tear would heal a lot better than a whacking great big cut with scissors!

It was also routine to shave a woman's pubic area before the birth. Not an easy task, as I'm sure most women will testify, and particularly irritating when the hair grows back. This is no longer deemed essential, thank goodness. Then an enema was administered with a jug of warm water, a funnel and a tube. The water was put into the woman's back passage, in order to clear out the bowel ready for the birth. Only when the bowel was full to bursting was the woman allowed to go to the toilet. Nowadays this procedure is felt to be unnecessary unless a woman is very constipated. And only a small sachet with a little nozzle is used which, although powerful, is more discreet. If anyone had peeped behind the bed curtains in the old days, they might have thought some weird scientific experiment was going on!

Since I hadn't been subjected to any of this nonsense when my children were born, I didn't agree with any of it. I'd had two natural births and my babies were fine, so I could see that these procedures weren't necessary. But there wasn't anything I could do about it. I just had to shut up and get on with it.

After my first delivery, I proudly boasted in the staff dining room that I had finally done it. 'You didn't keel over, then?' someone asked. But of course when I was doing, as opposed to just watching, I was perfectly all right.

Every birth I attended was an exhilarating experience for me. After the second delivery, one of the nursing officers who was supervising me asked me a couple of questions about the placenta, or afterbirth. I was so thrilled about the baby's birth that I couldn't remember a thing I'd been taught in class.

'You should be able to discuss the physiology of the placenta in detail now, Nurse,' she chastised. 'This is not good enough.'

She was quite hard on me really, but I was too ecstatic to care!

For a while, whenever I seemed to be making progress with my training and even becoming a little complacent, something always happened to jolt me down to earth again. One day I was looking after a woman in labour with her first baby and, as the birth was imminent, I called the midwife who was supervising me. She was rather an officious person and I didn't like her very much. When the baby was born I immediately saw that he had a harelip. This is an abnormality of the mouth which, although it appears quite shocking at first sight, is usually correctable. In this baby's case, after plastic surgery only a faint scar would remain.

To my horror, the midwife wrapped the baby up straight away and took him to the special care baby unit without saying a word to the parents. I was left to try and explain what the matter was with their son, as they had not been able to see his face. Quite soon after that, the midwife reappeared with the baby and a paediatrician and they all discussed the harelip. The parents were shocked and upset and were almost too frightened to look at their baby. I was left thinking how heartless the midwife had been and resolved never to behave in that way when I was qualified.

Happily, there was a wonderful midwife called Nora in charge of the labour ward. She was a lovely, plump, motherly Northern woman who was tremendously experienced and efficient, but also kind and compassionate. She made the junior doctors quake in their boots, because she was quite domineering and wouldn't suffer fools gladly. So she was nice to you if you were good, but if you were rubbish she would tell you so, however junior or senior you were.

In those days, the doctors learnt from the senior midwives. In theory they should have been learning from their senior colleagues, but the senior doctors frequently didn't bother to come and teach them. It was probably for the best, actually, because the senior midwives had the most experience, and in practice it was tacitly accepted that a senior midwife was more than qualified to teach a junior doctor.

Nora was so experienced that she would tell a doctor – any doctor, however senior – when she needed him to attend a birth with his forceps. 'Come along, dear,' she would say, and then guide him through the procedure. The doctors had to do the medical bits, but Nora could probably have done them better, as it happened. She bossed them around all the time.

'Get on with that!'

'Go and sew that woman up!'

'What are you doing that for? No, no, no!'

She knew just how to handle the more senior doctors, the registrars. If there was ever a problem, she would summon them and get them to do exactly what she wanted. They always complied. She also commanded the greatest respect from the often rather self-important consultants. Most importantly, the women loved her, as did the junior midwives. She taught them everything they needed to know and told them exactly what they had to do. I admired Nora so much and hoped to be just like her one day.

Often a midwife would come out of a labour room, sigh heavily and go and seek out Nora. 'Things are progressing really slowly, Sister, and I shall need to call the doctor for help if this woman doesn't deliver soon,' she'd say wearily.

'Go and make yourself a cup of tea and have yourself a break, love,' Nora would say. 'I'll take over for a few minutes.' After a short interval, she would appear at the door of the labour room with a baby in her arms, just in time to welcome the midwife back from her tea break. 'Shame you missed it, my love,' she'd say. 'It just happened so quickly at the end!'

None of us knew exactly what Nora did in that room to hasten the babies' arrival. She had all these little tricks of the trade. She always managed to get a baby out when you thought it wasn't going to come. She was an expert at gently inserting her fingers and turning the baby's head a bit or pushing it into place. I sometimes did this after I was qualified and it definitely works.

The cervix has to open up to ten centimetres before the birth happens and quite often a small part of it will wedge over the baby's head. Then the baby can't move and becomes distressed; it can be stuck for a few hours. Nora showed us how to push up the overlap part of the cervix and then ask the woman to push, so the baby's head could come down and bingo, out would come the baby. Techniques like that were invaluable.

She also taught us how to put women in different positions to dislodge their babies when they were stuck. She might put them on the bed with their knees drawn up to their chin, and it would make a real difference. It must have opened up the pelvis. I later learned that getting a woman to walk up and down stairs can really help, too. Something as simple as that can speed up labour by hours and even make the difference between having a caesarean and having a normal birth.

Nora would try lots of different things and it was fascinating to learn from her. You need somebody like that to teach you the skills they've picked up over the years. You always wondered what her trick had been if you weren't with her at a difficult delivery, when she somehow managed to perform her magic. Whatever it was, the mother always came out smiling!

* * *

There was a lovely doctor working on maternity at that time. His name was Mark and all the midwives fancied him – especially me. He was a real dreamboat with dark hair and big brown eyes, and the kind of smile that could melt you. One day he was in the operating theatre changing room, where all the doctors got into their green theatre tops and trousers ready for operating. A couple of the other students told me I was needed in there urgently, so I hurried in, only to find Mark in his underwear! Then the door suddenly locked behind me and I was trapped in there with him. Thanks girls! Mark wasn't a bit perturbed and just carried on changing, but I was weak at the knees and kind of lost my voice. Did I make the most of this golden opportunity? No, I just hammered on the door to be let out! Sadly, he was so good-looking that I knew I didn't have a hope in hell. The thought was nice, though.

I had one or two serious boyfriends over the course of my training. But I had to be careful because of the children; I didn't want them to get to know anybody unless he was going to be permanent. So it was more a case of making sure the children were being looked after and then going out and having fun. My fellow trainees and I had a great social life. Several of us used to go out in the evening together and sometimes we visited the local dance hall. When we met someone nice and they asked the predictable question about what we did for a living, their reactions to the answer were always amusing. It seems that only women who have had a baby are at ease talking to a midwife – and they usually just want to regale you with a blow-by-blow account of *all* their births, especially when you're off duty!

Men love meeting nurses, as they always conjure up visions from late-night movies with titles like *Naughty Night Nurses,* where women dressed in stockings and suspenders wander around brandishing thermometers. But midwives . . . no! It's a job title much more likely to elicit an image of a large lady with her hair in a bun driving a Morris Minor. Men have no idea what to say to a midwife at all – although one young man I met retaliated by telling me that he travelled in aluminium tubing. He wasn't a toothpaste salesman as I thought . . . but a pilot. He and I went out quite a bit and my mum definitely approved. 'Hang on to him!' she said. But there was something missing, somehow, and so I let him go.

Another good friend I made was a male student nurse called Geoff. I first met him at the hospital's outdoor swimming pool, where he was competently swimming length after length and I was . . . sunbathing. During the long, hot summer of 1976, I spent every lunchtime when I was at the hospital trying to get a suntan. I was always at the pool, but although I liked swimming, I never got wet! I only had three quarters of an hour for a break, so it was tanning only. Geoff, on the other hand, was super fit and loved sports. He mistakenly thought I was the sporty type because I was always at the pool, so when we started going out together I had to do all sorts of outdoorsy activities, like badminton and canoeing, before he realised that I was pretty hopeless at everything. However, we had lots of fun during our time at the hospital, until we went our separate ways when he failed his finals and left to join the Police Service.

Because I had been a mother from the age of nineteen,

I'd missed out on having a single girl's social life. Now I was enjoying making up for lost time with my new friends. My colleagues and I shared all the details of our personal lives with each other and never felt embarrassed about anything. When you're dealing with the basic facts of life, as we were every day, there's no room for shyness or inhibition. Dinner party conversations were often quite shocking for non-medical guests. We all gave each other lots of support during family crises or love-life problems and we made friendships that were to last a lifetime.

It was a time when social restrictions on women were beginning to relax. There was a real sense of freedom in the air for me, because I had been brought up by very Victorian parents. I never saw my parents without their clothes on and certainly nobody walked around naked. You never talked about anything to do with sex or babies, so I was having a ball now that everyone was opening up. It was great just to be able to talk about things openly and not have any embarrassment at all.

I remember sitting in a very boring lecture and discreetly taking out a book I had with me. It was called, *Now That You've Got Me Here, What Are You Going To Do?* and the author was a woman writing about her experiences with men in bed. I was riveted. 'Look at this!' I whispered to the pal next to me, showing her an extract under the desk. Neither of us raised our eyes from that book for the rest of the lecture!

4

Finding My Feet
1977

In my second year, when I was considered to be a senior student, I spent several very enjoyable weeks with a district midwife, now known as a community midwife, called Mrs Foord. We never used each other's Christian names, which seems unthinkable now. These days, patients, nurses and midwives are usually on first-name terms, and sometimes doctors are too, but thirty years ago it would have been considered disrespectful. I'm not sure that this new familiarity is always a good thing and certainly the older generation sometimes disapproves. I still think that when you are doing very intimate things for people, the dignity that comes from using their surname can be very welcome.

Mrs Foord ran antenatal clinics at a doctor's surgery, delivered babies at home and in hospital, and visited women at home after the birth. This was to be my chosen field. It didn't take long to confirm what I had suspected would be the case: I felt much more comfortable looking after women in the community and in their own homes than in hospital. All my instincts, as a mother and a midwife, were to aim for home births where it was safe to do so. It is inevitable that in hospital people become little more than a bed number or are known by the name of their particular condition, such as 'the breech in bed 3', rather than a person with hopes and fears and a home and family. I enjoyed getting to know the women in Mrs Foord's district and caring for them in pregnancy, labour and after the birth of their babies. It was much more satisfying than just meeting them for a short time in hospital.

I loved this part of my training and learnt such a lot from Mrs Foord. I can't say she became a friend, but she was kind to me and I respected her enormously. She had no children of her own, but enjoyed her work and the mothers trusted her judgement. I always met her at her house in the mornings before we began our day's work. She was a very religious woman. Her Bible was usually open on the kitchen table and she would often point out a passage or two to me; although I'd describe myself as an atheist, I tried to show interest in her beliefs.

We worked very hard and never finished our day's tasks until about two hours after the other midwives and their students, who considered 'the district' to be an easy option. Consequently they used to tease me and marvel at how I managed to cope with being with Mrs Foord for long stretches of time without using bad language! After all, it says in the Bible that one should not blaspheme, so I had to be very careful. The most I would ever have said is 'oh God!' or perhaps 'b****r!' but I managed to avoid even these.

Sometimes the district midwives had to be on call at night for women planning a home birth. Because I lived about fifteen miles away from the area we were covering, on those nights I stayed in a room in the nurses' home at the hospital. Sometimes it was two or three nights in a row and I didn't like it at all. The room was like a prison cell, very austere and sparsely furnished, and I wanted to be with my children. I was completely reliant on the support of my family to enable me to complete my training, and to have a social life as well as be a mother. My sister was an incredible help and looked after the boys frequently. I knew that they couldn't have been in safer hands than with my mother or sister, but still I fretted. I missed them.

On the very first night I was in the nurses' home, the telephone rang just after I had settled down on my own in the sitting room to watch television. It was Mrs Foord.

'Are you ready, Nurse?' she asked. 'We have a lady in labour.'

Ready? Definitely!

I was so excited; this was my first home birth. Would I be up to the job? It was so different from working in the hospital, where set procedures had to be followed at all times at a birth, where all the equipment had to be placed in exactly the right position on the trolley and the fetal heart monitor took up most of the room. In someone's home, it was more a case of having to improvise and making sure that everything needed was within reach.

I can see the point of having equipment in the same place in a hospital delivery room, because it makes it easier to find things in a hurry. But if there is no flexibility, and there definitely wasn't in those days, it's difficult to learn to think for yourself about the way you organise things. And in an unexpected situation, this makes you less confident and even a bit disorientated.

Everything went well at my first home birth with Mrs

Foord. It was so much more relaxed and intimate than the hospital births I had attended. It felt different in every way: even kneeling down beside the comfortable, homely, double bed was a sharp contrast to standing beside an impersonal, plastic-covered hospital delivery bed. Mrs Foord was kind and totally professional as usual and the mother seemed very calm; she was safe and secure in her family home. It felt very special to leave the house with mum, dad and new baby all happily snuggled in bed together. Even though I had given birth at home myself, I hadn't seen things from the midwife's point of view, so it was an excellent learning experience for me, and it confirmed everything I had previously believed about home births. I floated out of the house on an absolute high.

I felt fortunate that I had experienced childbirth before I began my training. It meant that I could really empathise with the women I was meeting. Even though I was a naive, terrified nineteen-year-old when I had Matthew, I had found it an exhilarating and empowering experience – once the midwife arrived! Then of course I had a planned home birth for my second child, Edward, in 1970. Both experiences strengthened my belief that childbirth should not be medicalised, unless for a very good reason.

Edward was born just before home birth started to be discouraged, so it was normal practice then. Then the Government's Peel Report in 1970 stated that provision should be made for all women to give birth in hospital, which gave people the idea that giving birth at home was dangerous. There was a huge shake-up in maternity services, so that whereas I saw the same local midwife all through the pregnancy and she came for the birth, this tended to happen less and less. It really doesn't happen very often now, except in a few enlightened areas of the country. Mostly women see a variety of midwives and are cared for in labour by a midwife they have never met before. Apparently, research has shown that women don't mind either way, but I wonder what questions were actually asked in the research – and how they were worded.

'Were you happy with the care you had?' This is a question which may well elicit positive responses, but what if it was put in a different way? 'Would you have preferred a midwife you knew?' Would the results be the same?

After my spell on the district, I was now absolutely convinced that community midwifery was the area in which I wanted to practise and I felt my training was really coming together. Back at the hospital, I had a spell in the antenatal ward, where women stayed if they had complications during pregnancy. In the 1970s it was more difficult to diagnose problems since we didn't have the benefit of all the technology available today. Women often spent weeks, even months, in hospital, which rarely seems to happen nowadays. Of course, these women got to know the midwives very well and when their story had a happy ending, all the staff were thrilled. One woman who had been trying to have a baby for many years spent about three months in the antenatal ward and when her daughter was born she very aptly named her Angel. It was so lovely to see her proudly cradling Angel, because she had been so desperate for a baby and virtually lost all hope of having one.

There were three consultant obstetricians on the ward who made frequent visits and often used the women for teaching purposes. The patients didn't object – they didn't dare. I grew used to seeing the consultants, usually accompanied by several terrified student midwives or medical students, stride up to a poor unsuspecting woman in her bed and bellow at her: 'You don't mind me discussing your case with these people, do you my dear?'

He would then completely ignore her and talk about all sorts of dreadful possible complications, and ask lots of questions that the students couldn't answer, before flouncing off to attack someone else!

The consultants' favourite trick was to catch the students out. They were often asked to examine a woman's abdomen and say which way the baby was lying; not always an easy task, even when you have experience. The consultant would always pick a woman who had twins or a baby who was in an unusual position, so that the student would be humiliated when they got it wrong – which they invariably did. Sometimes the woman would collude and try to mouth the right answer to the students and this always merited a special thankyou when the doctor had disappeared.

The pupil midwives had to practise teaching antenatal classes as part of their training, so we used the women in the antenatal ward as guinea pigs. Well, they were a captive audience and couldn't get away even if they wanted to! Hopefully, they learnt something of interest into the bargain.

The postnatal ward was where the mothers stayed after

they had given birth. It was run like an army camp and everything was done by the clock. Although it appeared to be very regimented, it did in fact run quite smoothly. Some postnatal wards these days appear to be a bit of a shambles, with visiting allowed all day and no rest time for the mothers. That wasn't a problem in the 1970s. But what did strike me as wrong was the way babies were treated. It didn't matter whether they were breast or bottle fed, they all stayed in the ward nursery and were allowed out only at feeding times. All babies had their feeds at the same time, at four-hourly intervals. The breastfed babies were given a small bottle of water to top them up after each feed, a practice deemed completely unnecessary and even harmful today. Then they went back to the nursery and their mums had a rest. Visitors were kept to a minimum and even fathers were only allowed to visit twice a day for an hour. Women stayed in hospital at least six days if they had given birth to their first baby. It seemed a sad way to begin family life.

The midwives went round the ward saying, 'Breast or bottle?' to the new mums. This was before breastfeeding was seen as the best option, as it is today. Most people decided what they were going to do before the baby was born. They generally had in their minds whether they were going to go for breast or bottle. Women didn't seem to have so much trouble with breastfeeding as they do now – if they wanted to do it, they got on with it; if not, they bottle fed. Nowadays it's talked about so much that people can easily get in a state about it. Not that I am saying breastfeeding is always easy. Sometimes it isn't, which can be a source of huge frustration and upset for mothers. But I think, as with most things in life, your expectations have a large part to play.

If a mother didn't know what she wanted to do, she'd usually be offered a bottle. Bottle feeding was seen to be easier and so it was frequently recommended. No-one explained why breastfeeding might be better, probably because we didn't have so much information then. So we went through a few years where bottle feeding was in and breast was out. Now it's gone the other way of course, and women are made to feel terrible if they don't breastfeed. We've gone from one extreme to the other. In the 1970s, all the bottles were left out on a big trolley for people to go and collect. Now they're hidden away and you have to ask for them – and you often don't get them, unless you really need them.

When I had Matthew and Edward, the GPs I saw afterwards said, 'You're not going to breastfeed, are you? Here, have some pills, dry it up.' They definitely didn't encourage you to breastfeed then, but I wanted to, partly because my mother had done it, but also because it felt so natural. Nevertheless, after a few weeks, I decided it was too difficult to carry on with and took the doctors' advice. You didn't get any help with breastfeeding then. Nowadays helping women to breastfeed is a big part of the midwife's postnatal care.

With Matthew, I got mastitis, an infection of the breast, after a few weeks. I was really sick, with a raging temperature. The midwife came round and said, 'You've got to stop breastfeeding.' I didn't question it, because I thought she knew best; I went on antibiotics and gave it up. Since then I've found out that you don't have to stop breastfeeding at all, but they didn't know that then.

With Edward, I breastfed until one day he was sick and I thought he was ill. The doctor came round and said, 'It's probably the breast milk. You're overfeeding him or something. I should put him on the bottle.' So I did. How pathetic! But I was just doing what I was told.

By the time I qualified as a midwife, my policy was that breastfeeding was best. I didn't insist on it; I just said, 'I'll help you if you want me to help you.' A lot of people were bottle feeding then, but I felt that breastfeeding was more natural and therefore better. There are advantages to the bottle: it's easier and the baby sleeps longer, but obviously it's not as good for the baby or the mum. Breastfeeding helps to prevent breast cancer and that's a huge thing. Still, we didn't know all of this in the 1970s.

If a baby had to stay in the special care baby unit, its mother was only allowed to visit in the morning and evening for ten minutes. I thought this was totally wrong. Surely a sick baby needs its parents even more than a healthy one! And the parents needed to spend time with their child in order to adjust to whatever problems they had. It seemed perfectly obvious to me, but not to the nursing officer in charge of the special care baby unit, sadly.

There were several reasons why babies were admitted to the unit. They may have been delivered with forceps or had jaundice or feeding difficulties. Some were small or premature and some were ill. I remember particularly a set of twins named Michael and Joseph. Michael was healthy and just a little small. Joseph however was very brain-damaged and was likely to need care for life, although it was impossible to determine exactly what his quality of life would be at that stage. The doctors could merely guess. The nursing officer took his parents aside and spoke to them quietly.

'Now my dears, wouldn't you prefer to take just one healthy baby home, instead of having the burden of a severely damaged child as well?'

The parents agreed that one healthy child would be a better option, although I don't know if that was truly their wish or whether they felt pressured into making the decision. Consequently Joseph was made comfortable and only given water until he eventually died. I am not sure if this was common practice at that time, but I think it happened more than we realised.

I used to feel very upset for the mothers whose babies were kept in the nursery and those whose babies were in special care. Because my babies were born at home, I knew the joy of having them next to me all the time and I know I would have reacted very badly if someone had taken them away from me. I loved watching them while they slept and talking to them when they were awake and making funny faces. Although I didn't know it at the time, this is part of the attachment process that bonds mother and child. I sensed through my own experience – and later learnt by reading up on psychological research – that this bonding paves the way for a good parent and child relationship in the future. I therefore decided that I must bring the matter up at one of our regular staff meetings at the hospital. I suggested that we should try to keep mothers and babies together as much as possible. It wasn't right to separate them.

Even when a baby was first born, it was taken to the nursery on the labour ward to be bathed and was left there alone until mum was washed and ready to go to the postnatal ward. I questioned the senior staff about this. 'How can a mother bond with her baby with these rules?'

I was told off in no uncertain terms!

'Nurse, you know this word "bonding" is a modern term with no meaning. What's more, you shouldn't believe everything you read in the papers.'

Well, at least I tried! I often used to question policies and practices which I found bizarre. I read anything I could get my hands on about childbirth. There weren't a lot of books around at the time, but I read everything in print by Sheila Kitzinger, Frederick Leboyer and Grantly Dick-Read, as well as midwifery journals and newspapers. I scoured the library and bookshops in my area; as time went on, my local second-hand bookshop began to stock a good collection of books about childbirth, because women don't keep them after they've read them. Eventually, I built up my own little library that I used to lend out to people.

Although I felt dissatisfaction with a lot of the procedures I was being trained to carry out, I often found myself in a dilemma: I was against the medicalisation of childbirth, but I was very loyal to the hospital and my colleagues. So when a complaint appeared in the local newspaper about the maternity department, my instinct was to defend it. A lady accused the midwives of being unkind to her daughter, who had recently given birth to her first baby. It may well have been true, but those of us who considered ourselves to be kind and caring were very offended. I therefore decided to compose a reply in verse defending the midwives. Of course, I asked permission before sending it to the newspaper and I was thrilled when it was published.

I practise as a midwife at the famous S and V
And things that Mrs Saunders said have really saddened me.
I greet my patients with a smile and put them at their ease,
I comfort them and ease their pain and try so hard to please.
I like to have the dads around, to them I'm never rude
And if I ever send them home, it's just to have some food.
And when at last the baby lies in mother's arms I'm glad,
Then I wrap him up quite tightly and give him to his dad.
So please don't think we're all like Sarah Gamp at the S and V,
Because I really love my work and there's lots more here like me!

Sarah Gamp was a fictional character from a Charles Dickens novel. She was an alcoholic nurse/midwife who was a disgrace to the profession.

The lady then replied to me in verse and this was also published in the local paper.

IT'S NO RUMOUR – A NURSE WITH HUMOUR

Thank you for the charming verse from Agnes Light
* – nurse.*
It serves to quash the nasty rumour that midwives
* lack a sense of humour*
Faith that this darling's one of many, sir I really
* haven't any.*
Nightingales of veil and lamp are still outnumbered
* by S. Gamp.*
May we hope that this sweet dreamer persuades
* those nurses who grow meaner,*
That they could get their just desserts when they feel
* blue and when it hurts.*
One day it might be their lot to need a hand around
* the cot.*
If they should I hope their nurse is just like them – or
* even worse!*

I didn't think it wise to continue this rhyming discourse, as it might have gone on forever!

There was a different atmosphere in the hospital at night. All the students had to work on night duty for a few weeks at a time and during my time on nights I grew certain that more women begin labour at night than during the day. Maybe this is because their bodies are winding down and relaxing, so the uterus feels a burst of energy and gets on with it. One doctor believed it had something to do with the rhythms of Earth and the Moon and he was planning to conduct research into his theory, but I thought it was more likely to be related to hormones or a woman's body clock. Also, babies are nocturnal; they're like hamsters. After they're born, they're usually awake all night.

There were fewer medical staff around at night and a kind of calm descended on the labour ward, even though babies continued to be born through until dawn. We senior students were given a bit more responsibility now and two of us were sometimes allowed to deliver a baby together, without the supervision of a qualified midwife. By now, we had all delivered countless babies, albeit with a qualified midwife on hand, but heaven knows what the mothers would have thought if they had known we weren't actually qualified! We didn't tell them of course, and there were so many different types of uniform that they never knew who was who. In fact my friend Jenny, a mere student at the time, was once addressed by a mother as 'Matron' and Jenny was so flattered she didn't correct her! Doctors were so revered in those days that people rarely asked medical professionals to identify themselves when they entered their room. Anyone wearing a white coat could walk in, examine them and walk out without being questioned. People were too trusting then, but thankfully things have changed now.

In the early hours of the morning one of the treasured auxiliary nurses wheeled a clanking old trolley into the office. It was groaning under the weight of a huge pot of tea and a mountain of hot buttered toast that was always gratefully pounced on by the midwives. You were always really pleased if you managed to get back into the office for the toast round, because you feel at your lowest ebb between three and four o'clock in the morning. Your blood sugar drops and you need the toast as a pick-me-up. Years later it still tastes heavenly after a difficult night shift.

When the toast arrived, we had the chance to discuss what was happening in the ward and whether there had been any emergencies. We often had a chuckle, too: 'Did you see that woman's husband? Wasn't he ghastly?' If it was quiet, then we'd talk about other things: our children or our dogs. Tired as we were, we never seemed to run out of conversation. We had been training together for more than a year and were now a close-knit group.

As senior students, we had to learn how to be the scrub midwife in the operating theatre. After getting scrubbed up – in other words, changing into a green theatre top and trousers, washing our hands thoroughly and donning a sterile theatre gown and gloves – the job of the scrub midwife was to set out the surgical instruments on a trolley in the correct order, ready for use. Some obstetric surgeons have been known to shout and throw things if they are handed the wrong instrument, so I was not looking forward to this part of the training! I was quite scared of making a mistake and showing myself up. However, I managed quite well, and while I was still a student there was always a qualified midwife there to help out. I also decided that I would retaliate if I was shouted at. I was a mature adult and a mother and as such I deserved politeness.

There have been only two occasions during my career when I have encountered outright rudeness from doctors. Each time I quietly and firmly confronted the doctor involved afterwards and asked him (it was always a him!) not to speak to me like that again, particularly in front of patients or other staff. The doctors apologised and treated me charmingly afterwards. I don't think it is necessary to be rude or shout in order to get people to do what you want. Everyone deserves courtesy and respect no matter what their job or their status.

Another thing that we had to learn about was suturing, or stitching, a woman's perineum after birth. As I've already said, the perineum may be damaged when the baby's head emerges, so it's very important for the mother's future comfort and sex life that the suturing is done competently. After bad suturing, some women suffer great pain and are unable to walk or sit comfortably for many months, so I felt it was a huge responsibility.

Never having been able to sew or knit, I feared I might not get the hang of it. I vaguely recall going to sewing lessons at school, but I can't have been very interested in them, because now I kept hearing people talk about blanket stitch and I hadn't the faintest clue what it was! 'Practice makes perfect' is the saying, but who wants to be practised on? No-one, surely! This was another occasion when it was reassuring to have a qualified midwife looking over your shoulder, ready to step in should you need a hand.

In the 1970s, the doctors were the ones who did most of the suturing. One day, a young doctor took me outside the room and said, 'I've never sewn anybody up. Can you show me how to do it?'

'Oh dear, it's like the blind leading the blind!' I thought.

'You'd better phone the registrar to come and help you,' I advised. What would the woman inside the room have said if she'd overheard our conversation? I dread to think. Fortunately, I gradually gained experience of suturing and learnt how to do it well – and by the 1980s it was decided that midwives should do it instead of doctors. Since midwives are probably more aware of the potentially agonising consequences of bad stitching than the doctors are, because they are more involved with after-birth care, I think it's a good thing that they took over the suturing.

Another department where senior students had to gain experience was the special care baby unit (SCBU), more commonly known as 'skaboo' among the nurses and medical staff. I was always nervous about working in this area, because the babies were usually small and vulnerable and needed expert care. As a midwife you get used to working in situations where one slip or lapse of concentration can mean the difference between everything running smoothly and a potentially risky situation for mother or baby. I was developing the ability to keep calm under pressure but there was something especially nerve-racking about working with these tiny poorly babies. The emotional turmoil could be overwhelming if you weren't careful. And of course, a flustered midwife is not a useful midwife. Our job was to observe, listen and learn. It was vital that medicines were carefully checked for the correct dosage; getting the dosage even slightly wrong could be disastrous for such fragile patients.

I felt sad for the parents, as they were rarely allowed to get involved in their baby's care – and sometimes they were too scared. It was especially upsetting when the procedures made their infant cry. It must have been so difficult for them. They had to put their trust in strangers to do the best they could for their beloved child. After every shift in the special care unit I would heave a sigh of relief and thank my lucky stars, again, for my two beautiful healthy boys.

Babies were admitted to the unit for what would be considered unnecessary reasons today, such as newborn jaundice, which can be managed on the postnatal ward. Jaundice can be serious if it's severe, but usually it isn't. It was awful that the parents of babies with mild jaundice could only go down to special care at eleven o'clock and five o'clock, so they only got to see their babies twice a day. It was totally unnecessary for them to be so restricted. Every baby who'd been delivered with forceps was also in special care, which doesn't happen anymore. Of course, they don't use forceps very often now, preferring to use the ventouse – a kind of suction cup device which fits onto the baby's head and helps the doctor guide the baby out while the mother pushes – but either way, the forceps babies did not need to be in SCBU.

Weeping mothers were a common sight and I felt so sorry for them. I couldn't tell them that I didn't agree with the policy of separating them from their babies, because that would have been unprofessional, but I used to try and comfort them. All our hearts went out to them and we spent as much time as we could sitting with them and talking, so that they weren't just sitting on their own. All around them were mothers who were feeding their babies. It was so cruel!

I don't think the people in charge realised just how terrible it is to have a baby taken away from you. It leaves you feeling completely bereft. The three spinsters that ran the place were devoted nurses, but they had very little compassion when it came to this issue. I'm not saying you have to have children to understand the pain the mothers were feeling; I think it would have been possible for anyone to empathise. But for some reason these women had completely closed minds. They never used to listen to what people said. They just thought that things had to be done properly, to the book, according to national policy, and they wouldn't deviate from that at all. It was hard not to resent them for it.

These days, because of advances in technology, babies survive after fewer weeks in the womb than they used to in the 1970s. Pregnancy normally lasts for forty weeks, but babies born at twenty-two weeks may now be kept alive. Therefore there are more very premature and seriously ill babies needing specialised care in neonatal intensive care units than ever before. Some people think it is wrong to keep babies alive if they are born much too early, because they frequently suffer from disabilities, and of course there are cost implications too. But how can doctors decide not to treat them when the technology is available? And who should decide whether a child lives or dies? It is easy to make sweeping statements about what should or should not happen when you are not the parent involved. But it can be almost impossible to predict the quality of life a child might come to have since the extent of their disability often cannot be determined at birth. Our stint at the special care baby unit proved to be a challenging one for us students, but rewarding too, when we saw babies finally go home with their parents.

I had the chance to become adept at catching babies when I did a spell with the community midwives in my second year. The community midwives were always a lovely motherly group of women who gave you bags of confidence and passed on all their little tricks. This was when it became really clear to me for the first time what I was supposed to be doing with my hands. 'You put your hands there and I'll do the talking,' one of the midwives directed.

She was watching very carefully and saying to the woman, 'Now push, now pant, now push again,' and to my amazement I could feel the response to what she was saying.

'Now I understand!' I thought.

Some people are definitely better at teaching than others. Many of the other midwives I assisted just let me get on with it – and if I made a complete mess of it, well, too bad.

* * *

Soon it was time for my final exams and one of these was an oral test, or viva, which took place in London. This was a terrifying experience for some of the students. We travelled to our destination by train and spent the journey making each other more and more nervous. We were then in a highly charged, anxious state on arrival. The oral examination was to take place in a rather old and imposing building belonging to the Royal College of Midwives in Mansfield Street. It had probably been a very grand Victorian terraced house in the past. There was a sign above the doorway in Latin which read: 'Abandon all hope ye who enter here', a quote from Dante's *Inferno*, warning visitors at the gates of hell. The mind boggles as to why it was up there, but it was strangely applicable to us that day!

Inside, the building was filled with pupil midwives from all over the country looking intimidated and whispering nervously to each other. I felt strangely calm though. I had decided that if I failed to qualify it would not be the worst thing to happen. I wasn't totally focused on my career; my children were the most important part of my life and I was in the process of divorcing my husband at the time. I had more significant and stressful things to worry about.

The viva was set to last about fifteen minutes and the questions could be about any topic. There were several eminent doctors sitting around a large room behind small individual tables, each with an empty chair for the 'victim'. Several students could thus be tested at the same time. I was soon called in to meet my examiner. He was a rather kind senior obstetrician who tried to put me at ease.

Unfortunately, I had no idea how to answer his first question. 'What would you do to find out if someone had a urine infection if the pathology laboratory were shut?' he asked.

I apologised and said I didn't know. 'You would look at it under a microscope to see if there were bacteria present,' he said. I thanked him for giving me the answer, while secretly thinking, 'Where would I find a microscope on the ward?'

I managed to answer the rest of the questions, but was convinced my first mistake would count against me. I felt quite dejected on the train journey home, which was a pity because everyone else was obviously relieved it was over and the atmosphere was very jolly. Meanwhile, I stared disconsolately out of the train window, thinking about how I couldn't qualify as a midwife without passing the viva. And after all that work, too.

I did my best to distract myself while I waited for the letter to come with my results. I had pretty much got to the point of believing that I genuinely had no chance of qualifying, and was mentally preparing for the fact that my long-cherished, much-delayed dream had gone down the tubes again. So imagine my surprise when a letter came congratulating me on my success. The feeling was incredible. As soon as I opened that letter and saw the words telling me I'd passed, I realised I had been fooling myself when I tried to pretend I wouldn't have minded failing the viva. But fortunately, now I could just relax and celebrate. In fact, almost everyone from our group passed, and we certainly celebrated in style! When the Award

Presentation Day came I was so thrilled. I had started training to be a nurse at age eighteen and now I finally had a professional qualification, at the age of twenty-nine.

I had not forgotten how much I had disappointed my parents when I was younger, so it was lovely to be able to invite them to my qualifying ceremony. I was pleased they could be proud of my achievement at last – and they were absolutely delighted. There were tears in their eyes at the ceremony and my mother couldn't stop telling everybody that her daughter was now a midwife. My dad didn't ever express a lot of emotion, but it was obvious he was very proud. 'Don't you think she's done well?' he said to one of the tutors after the ceremony. 'She's got two children, you know, and she's managed to do all this training.'

'Listen to you!' I thought, remembering how he had chucked me out of home a decade before.

It was a really big deal to finally have my parents' approval. I felt vindicated; I had done the right thing at last. Life had come full circle and I'd made it, despite everything. I felt that I had become a person in my own right. I wasn't just a mother; I also had a career, and that meant such a lot to me.

Although our relationship hadn't always been easy, I forgave my father, because I knew he would have done anything for my children and me. I knew he cared very much; he just wasn't good at expressing emotion and had found it very hard to cope with the fact that I'd let him down. I think that was characteristic of his generation, and his alcoholism didn't help. I don't think any of us understood what the disease was about at the time, or even that it was a disease. Now everybody knows that alcoholism is an illness that's very hard to treat, but back then it was something that just wasn't talked about, along with so many other difficult subjects.

My only worry now was finding a job. It's hard to imagine in today's climate – where there's a chronic shortage of midwives – but back in 1978 there was a surplus of midwives and nurses and the training hospital was under no obligation to employ me after I qualified, especially as I had been a somewhat rebellious student! But I was desperate to get out there and put all that training to good use, and of course I needed to work to pay the bills.

As my boys were still quite young, I wanted to work part-time and avoid inconvenient shifts so that I could be with them as much as possible. Fortunately, while I was training I'd had a huge amount of support from my family, who lived close by. The children were always cared for by their auntie or grandma and seemed to adapt well to my strange working hours. I spent all my off-duty time entertaining them. They also remained close to their father and his family, which gave them extra stability, and I maintained a friendly relationship with the ex-in-laws too. It made life easier all round.

I have never understood why some people cut themselves off from their partner's family after they split up. It often seems like the children are being used as a weapon, which might be tempting when there's a lot of bad feeling, but is likely to be damaging for everyone involved. Grandparents bring an extra dimension to family life, as

well as helping with childcare and often with material
necessities. We never had a lot of money, but we had a
comfortable home, and with both families helping out we
managed well on my student's salary. I consider myself to
have been quite well off compared to student nurses and
midwives today. Now that their training is university
based, they receive a grant or a bursary that amounts to
much less than the salary I earned as a student.

I hardly dared hope that there would be a part-time
post available, as working full-time was the norm for
midwives back then. I made enquiries at my local hospital,
but had no luck. So then I decided to try my training
hospital, even though it meant continuing to travel fifteen
miles to work and back again. However, with my reputation for outspokenness I feared the worst. My card was
undoubtedly marked by many of the sisters in the hospital
because I was always asking questions and disagreeing
with policy. Worst of all was the ghastly sister who had
told me off for being too nice to people.

I faced the fearsome boss with trepidation. She was the
most senior – and intimidating – of the three spinsters. 'I
don't suppose you have a job for me?' I asked glumly.

To my amazement, she flashed me a broad smile.
'Actually, I can offer you three days a week in the labour
ward, if it suits,' she said briskly.

Well, I was gobsmacked! Had I been wrong about my
difficult reputation? Or did she just think I could be an
asset, once I'd been persuaded to keep my mouth shut and
not rock the boat too much? I knew that the sister had
been very pleased with me when I'd written the poem

defending midwives; she'd thought it was a good advert for the hospital. So maybe that was it!

Anyway, once I'd got over my surprise and elation, I began to look forward to the prospect of taking up my new job as a qualified midwife. However, I couldn't help feeling a little apprehensive too. After all, I wouldn't be a student anymore, with constant supervision. This time I was going to be in charge.

5

Qualified at Last!
1978

On my first day in my new role, I was allocated a student midwife to teach. There is a saying in the National Health Service that is usually applied to doctors: 'See one, do one, teach one!' Now it applied to me. It was terrifying. I'd finished my training, qualified, got a job and now I'd been given my own pupil on my very first day at work. There was no mentoring, no support, nothing; it was simply a case of: 'You're a midwife now; get on with it.' It wasn't heart surgery, but it was a huge responsibility to start teaching someone else. I was worried that I wouldn't be an adequate teacher, because I was so new to the job myself. But that's how it works in the NHS and there was nothing I could do to change it.

During the first week, I was in charge of the small unit attached to the labour ward, where each day women arrived for their labour to be induced or started off. Induction was carried out usually because the pregnancy had lasted twelve days after the due date. Some of the women mistakenly called it inducement, which makes it sound like there would be some sort of enticement or treat. But this procedure certainly wasn't any fun.

After her obligatory shave and enema, each woman was

given a tablet called pitocin, which contained a hormone that was supposed to soften up the neck of the womb. Before it was discovered in the 1950s, some midwives say they used castor oil for the same purpose. In fact the women were given the OBE . . . oil, bath and enema. After the tablet came the final attack: a vaginal examination where the bag of water was broken with an instrument like a pair of long-handled scissors. Then, if necessary, an intravenous drip containing a hormone was administered to finish the job off.

On one occasion I had six women in the unit for induction. After I had carried out all the shaves and enemas, which had taken me the whole morning, I was told that because the labour ward was so busy, the women could not be started off that day and they would have to go home. Well, none of us took that news very well, especially as the women had to come back for a repeat session the following day. Being a midwife was full of these frustrations and hold-ups. As well as coping with the highs and lows, I had to learn how to be patient when babies, or duty managers, took their time over things.

Very soon after I started, I delivered a baby that had a harelip. Mindful of how callously the midwife in charge had dealt with this situation the last time I had seen it happen, I slowly and carefully wrapped the baby up, while asking the parents if they knew what a harelip was. I gently explained the problem to them, told them their baby was still beautiful and would need their love and support. When I placed the baby in her mother's arms, she told the child how much she was loved and wanted. The father then cuddled both his wife and the baby and I knew they would cope with whatever lay ahead. After tidying up and reassuring the parents as much as possible, I asked the paediatrician to talk to them. I then helped the student I was supervising to come to terms with what had happened, as it is a shock for everyone when a baby is born with a disability. It was a sad moment for the parents in some ways, but I did my best to help everyone remember what was important: the birth of a much-loved and otherwise healthy baby. These are the times in which your skill as a midwife can really make a difference to people's lives and I left work that day feeling a huge amount of satisfaction, my heart full of quiet confidence that the family would cope.

The second week on duty started and, just my luck, we had a Flying Squad call. This meant there was an emergency situation somewhere in our area and either the woman, her family, the general practitioner or the district midwife had called for help. The Flying Squad comprised an ambulance containing two personnel and was dispatched to the hospital from the ambulance station. On arrival, a doctor and a midwife joined the crew, taking with them a special pack of emergency obstetric equipment. This included blood for a transfusion, if needed, and a portable baby incubator. Sometimes an obstetric doctor specialising in maternity care was required and sometimes a paediatric or children's doctor, if the patient was a newborn baby. We didn't always know exactly what the emergency was when the call came through to the labour ward, so it was quite frightening to be sent to accompany the doctor. Often it was only on arrival at the house, supermarket or airport – or wherever the situation was unfolding – that the problem was ascertained. A mother could be bleeding heavily before or after a home birth, or a woman planning a hospital delivery might be experiencing a rapid labour and was about to give birth unattended.

Whenever the Flying Squad was summoned, there was a mass exodus to the toilets by any junior midwives not busy with women in labour! We preferred to let the senior midwives go. But being new and unused to this event, I found myself the only person around when one particular emergency call came through. So naturally I was sent to accompany the doctor.

Fortunately, the problem wasn't too serious: a mother who was about to give birth at home unattended. By the time we arrived at the house, the baby had been born. Ambulance control was in telephone contact with the father, giving him detailed instructions about what to do, and they relayed the developments to us while we were racing to our destination.

Hurtling along the road with a blue light flashing and a siren howling, it was impossible to keep calm and think rationally. The adrenalin was pumping when we finally screeched to a halt. We all ran up the driveway and in through the open front door, where we were ushered into a bedroom by a woman who was either a relative or a neighbour. It was impossible to know, as the house was full of people chattering excitedly.

'The midwife's here, everyone! Thank goodness!' a voice shouted.

I was in such a hyped-up state that I thought, 'Oh good, the panic's over.' Then I suddenly realised . . . the midwife was me!

I somehow managed to pretend that I was actually in control and knew what I was doing, even though I felt out of my depth. Let's face it, I had some experience of home births, but it was nothing compared to the number of hospital births I'd attended. Fortunately, reinforcements soon arrived in the form of the local district midwife, who took over with bustling efficiency. I returned to the hospital with the doctor and ambulance crew expecting a hero's welcome. Far from it.

'Oh there you are at last,' the sister said in an exasperated tone. 'We've got very busy since you left; there's a patient in room five for you to look after.'

After that, I learned to hide in the toilets when the Flying Squad called. It was like some bizarre kind of initiation ceremony for the newest member of staff. However, I did make a point of asking one of the tutors how to cope with emergency childbirth, in case I was ever caught out again. Since then I've been desperate to be on an aeroplane and to hear the captain put a call out to the passengers: 'Is there a midwife on board, please?' Sadly this hasn't yet happened!

My three days a week were always very busy, exciting days. Although it was sometimes tiring, we all worked as a team. We newly qualified midwives went out together occasionally in the evening and had a lot of fun. It was necessary to let your hair down sometimes to compensate for working in a very emotionally demanding profession. After all, there wasn't always a happy outcome to childbirth.

I particularly remember a lady called Mary who gave birth prematurely to triplets who all died. She gave birth normally as the babies were too young to live anyway and the doctor felt a caesarean section would cause her more distress. Before epidural anaesthesia was so widely available, women were given a general anaesthetic if they needed a caesarean delivery. There were obviously risks associated with this and it was generally avoided if possible. Now, in the twenty-first century, many women choose to avoid a normal vaginal delivery for numerous reasons and epidurals are frequently given, especially for caesarean sections.

Mary had strong pain-relieving drugs during labour, in order that she should suffer as little as possible. Some people think a caesarean section would be quicker and easier when a baby is not expected to survive, but the general thinking is that it is cruel to leave a mother with a scar that will always remind her of the traumatic event. It may also mean that she has to undergo a caesarean next time. It takes longer to recover from the operation than is generally thought and there are associated risks, such as infection.

I never found out whether poor Mary and her husband were able to have another child. Sometimes it is hard to meet people in the middle of a crisis in their lives and then never see them again. We always like to believe there is a happy ending.

Another lady called Pamela had a sad tale to tell. She and her husband had been trying for ten years for a baby.

The strain of all the tests and years of anxiety became too much for their marriage to survive and they separated. Then Pamela found out shortly after the split that she was pregnant. I met her when she came into hospital in the early stages of labour. She had brought a little cassette player with her so that she could listen to her favourite music. She had no-one to accompany her, as her husband had met another woman and although he knew about the baby, he chose not to be with her for the birth. As she told me her story, we listened to Rose Royce singing, 'You abandoned me, love don't live here anymore.' I felt so sad for this brave lady. Although excited about the forthcoming birth, she missed her husband very much. I think of her whenever I hear that song and hope that they were eventually reunited.

One young girl who came into the hospital in labour caused some consternation among the staff. Paula had been married for about a year and had suffered from a condition that meant she was unable to consummate the marriage. I only found this out when I asked her permission to perform an internal examination. I needed to see how labour was progressing and find out the position of the baby.

'I'm sorry, I don't think you'll be able to,' she whispered.

When touched, her vagina invariably became very tense and went into a spasm, so examining her was out of the question. Amazingly, she had become pregnant when her husband had ejaculated outside her vagina. I consulted with the doctor, who was very kind and sympathetic to her, but to no avail. She became hysterical at the thought of being examined. She eventually had to have a general anaesthetic and a forceps delivery as it was the only way the baby could be delivered. Even though she must have been terrified about the birth, she had kept her secret throughout her pregnancy. I wondered if the poor girl had been subjected to abuse as a child, or whether in fact she had a purely physical problem. It was arranged for her and her husband to have counselling after she went home. I hope it was successful.

I have seen several stillbirths during my career. The first time was soon after I qualified. The mother was not my patient, but I was informed that she did not wish to see her dead baby. We have since learnt that this is not the best way to help a parent to grieve the loss of a newborn. Nowadays, the baby stays with the parents for as long as they wish and will be bathed and dressed and treated with the same care as a living baby. On this day, the baby was left in a small room near where the mother was recovering after the birth. I went to look at it, wanting to pay my respects in some way, and feeling that it was something I must be able to face.

There was a medical student working on the labour ward that day and I found him in the room practising intubation on the baby. This involves inserting a tube into the airway and is a procedure that may need to be done in an emergency to save a baby's life. I felt quite shocked when I saw what he was doing.

'Look, it's difficult for doctors to get the required expertise unless we can practise on dead bodies,' he explained. Of course, I knew that medical students did a lot of experiments on corpses; it was part of their training. 'You really should do it, too,' he went on, 'so you can learn how.'

He persuaded me to try, although I really didn't want to. Were we right or wrong to do so? I don't know. I know the baby was beautiful and we treated her with care and respect. I hoped that I would never need to resuscitate a baby, but now felt confident that I would manage this tricky procedure if the occasion arose, so maybe we were justified. I've seen doctors and midwives trying to resuscitate babies in very serious circumstances. It's a horrible situation to be in, but one in which you must know what you're doing if you want to react quickly and safely. However, I still think of that little baby girl and her poor parents, and can't help feeling that it would have been better for them to have seen their child.

During the time I worked on the labour ward, my friend Jenny was working in the SCBU. Like me, she had been a very outspoken student. This was probably because we were both mature students and mothers, with a wealth of life experience to bring to our training. We both thought certain practices should be changed and often tried unsuccessfully to convince our superiors.

One day Jenny was feeling very jolly and decided to entertain the babies by singing to them. Instead of a lullaby, she chose 'Rivers of Babylon' by Boney M, which she performed with gusto, dancing and quite a bit of talent! Unfortunately, the fearsome nursing officer in charge of the SCBU unit chose that moment to visit and she was absolutely horrified by the scene. She immediately sent Jenny to the Chief Nursing Officer for a telling-off for her unprofessional behaviour.

If only the babies could have spoken in her defence, I'm sure they would have done so. Jenny, for her part, was absolutely disgusted to be treated like a naughty schoolgirl being sent to the headmistress, and she immediately resigned. This was a great loss to the unit, as she was a valuable member of the team. Happily, she found another job straight away and was very happy in it. And I reckon she continued to serenade the babies with Boney M hits!

Soon after this, I received my own dressing-down – quite unfairly, I thought. The source of the mix-up was fairly minor. When instruments were used in the course of a delivery, they were washed and sent back to the sterilising department in a paper bag. One day, a student midwife had used a pair of scissors that she thought were blunt and she had written a note on the outside of the bag to this effect. The bags had to be signed by the person who had used the instruments and students were not allowed to sign anything on their own, so I also signed the bag. Consequently, when I was next on duty, I was summoned to the Chief Nursing Officer's room. She said the proper procedure had not been followed. Instead of writing on the bag, I should have informed my superior, who would have sent a form to the sterilising department to inform them about the blunt scissors. I was to be given a formal written warning and this would go on my record.

Well, my friends from outside the NHS were outraged at this pettiness. 'I can't believe you put up with this treatment! Why are you working for such an organisation?' one of them exclaimed.

I began to wonder myself and decided there and then to investigate jobs elsewhere. I would try my local hospital again to see if they now had vacancies. I was still absolutely committed to my work and to the NHS, but I needed a change of environment.

While I was making enquiries, I was transferred to the antenatal clinic in the hospital. It was common practice for midwives to be rotated to all areas so that they became competent and confident in each department. I loved working in this area, as it is usually the first point of contact pregnant women have with a midwife and the system of care. It was a great opportunity to give them a good first impression.

I was a bit disappointed to find that, sadly, that opportunity was still being squandered far too often. It was just like the production line I remembered from my training days. There were still huge numbers of women attending the clinic unnecessarily and routinely seeing the consultant obstetricians for a few minutes only. I tried to be friendly and make each woman feel special, remembering how nervous I had been in the same situation, and I hope it made a difference. Nowadays it is generally accepted that low-risk women, those without complications, should see a midwife throughout the pregnancy. Only women who are deemed high-risk because of medical or pregnancy complications see the consultants. This means all women have more appropriate care, with more time for discussions if needed. When you've been a midwife for thirty years and seen so many changes, many of them for the worse, it can be hard to remember that some things really have improved. But I've no doubt that this is one of those areas: antenatal care is genuinely better, more sensitive and personalised now than it was, for both patients and staff.

The midwifery sister who had reported me to my tutor for being too friendly with the women was still in charge. Although she remained stern and authoritarian and I never came to like her, we managed to work together. Little did I know that we were destined to meet again years later when I became an independent midwife . . . and then I would have the upper hand!

To my delight, it wasn't long before I found out that there were vacancies for midwives at my local hospital. After a successful interview, I was lucky to be offered a part-time job there. I was a little bit sorry to leave my training hospital and all the friends I had made, but at the same time I was looking forward to working at a small maternity unit, where my role would be quite different – and challenging in ways I could not have envisaged.

6

Home Turf
1979

And so I started my new job at the hospital in my home
town. At last, travelling to work would be easier and I
would have more time with my children. They were nine
and ten by now, and typically boisterous schoolboys who
loved football and wore me out with their endless energy. I
adored them; they were the anchor in my life and never
failed to make me laugh, even after a long shift. Although
it was tough at times being a single mother with a busy,
demanding job, I wouldn't have changed anything.

The maternity unit was run by three ladies of a mature
age. As was often the case in the 1970s, they were spinsters
who had dedicated their lives to the NHS. Or, perhaps like
the midwives at my previous hospital, they had had fiancés
at one time in their lives, but had never married. Although
they had no children, these women were compassionate
and caring and were excellent at their jobs. One was
responsible for the running of the unit, another was in
charge during the night shifts and the third ran the SCBU.

My first encounter with the nursing officer (they are
now known as department managers and modern
matrons) who ran the maternity unit took place soon after
I began my first shift. I was wandering around trying to

memorise where the fire exits and toilets were located when I put my head round the door of one of the delivery rooms. There was Miss Griffiths with her sleeves rolled up, mopping the floor. I reeled with shock and hastily offered to take over the job.

'Certainly not!' she said with a grin. 'I am just as capable of mopping the floor as you are, Nurse!'

I hadn't encountered this sort of attitude at my training hospital. If a nursing officer met you in the corridor there, she would barely acknowledge you, let alone roll up her sleeves and start cleaning up when she could just tell you to do it instead. I had the utmost respect for Miss Griffiths after that. She was serene like a nun and so wise. Later, when I knew her better, I always felt I could go to her with a work-related or personal problem, and she would always come up with a solution, without being judgemental.

When Christmas came, six months after I started working at the hospital, Miss Griffiths telephoned me on Christmas morning and wished me a Happy Christmas.

'If you and the children are alone today, you would be most welcome to come into the unit to join us for Christmas lunch,' she said kindly.

All patients who were fit and able were sent home at Christmas, but there were a few who had to remain in hospital. It was traditional for the staff and patients to enjoy a meal together and the patients' families were also invited to join them. Sometimes the staff invited their families too, if they wished. Knowing that I was a single parent, dear Miss Griffiths had taken the time to telephone me, despite being busy organising the festivities and knitting tiny stockings to hang on the babies' cots. I was very touched. As it happened, I was busy entertaining my parents and other members of the family, but I never forgot her kind gesture.

I would have done anything to help Miss Griffiths after that. If she needed me to work an extra shift or bake cakes for a fundraising event, I happily helped out. Sadly, the NHS is no longer an institution that cares for patients and staff alike in this way. With the advent of more managers and administrators, the personal touch and the loyalty have all but gone.

As in every place I ever worked, the midwives at the hospital worked hard, socialised together and supported each other. I made some very good friends there who are still friends more than thirty years later. I think part of the reason for these long-lasting friendships, the most solid of my career, was that we were working in one of the remaining small units, where we really had time to get to know each other and, more importantly, the women and their families. There were about a thousand babies born at the maternity unit each year, a quarter of the number born at my training hospital. The Government decided to phase out these small maternity units in the 1980s in favour of larger, better equipped and better staffed maternity units, where about five or six thousand babies a year would be born. Of course, progress needs to be made, the NHS needs to move forward, and change can improve things. But if I have learnt anything over the course of my career, it is that childbirth should not be medicalised for all women. The smaller units can often provide a better experience and they have a proven safety record.

During my first week, I was put in charge of the postnatal ward. This was a truly terrifying moment. I had never run a ward before – or written a report on patients or conducted a medicine round – and I soon realised that my training had not equipped me for these new challenges. If I had qualified as a nurse first, I would probably have felt a lot more confident, and for the first time I felt inferior to the other midwives, who were all trained nurses.

I had anticipated this problem while I was a student. 'Do you think the fact that I am not a nurse will be an obstacle in my career?' I had asked one of my tutors.

'It won't matter at all,' she assured me. 'If you have a patient with a medical condition you haven't come across, I'm confident in your abilities to research it thoroughly. Some girls just do the midwifery course to get an extra qualification that they may never use, whereas I know your heart is truly in midwifery.'

Her words had reassured me then . . . but now it didn't seem so simple. Well, here I was and I just had to get on with it. I blundered through the day and fortunately no-one came to any harm, but I had never felt so edgy on the job.

A very charming doctor arrived ten minutes after I started the shift and asked to see the newly admitted antenatal patients. 'Look, Doctor,' I told him, 'I've only just found the office, the telephone and the toilet; I haven't found the patients yet, so can you go on your own, please?'

And he did! Lionel was a wonderful doctor, as I soon found out. Some months later, I was working on the labour ward when I accompanied a lady into the operating theatre for an emergency caesarean section. Unfortunately, Lionel's junior doctor was nowhere to be found, so he asked me to take his place.

'Don't worry,' he said, 'I'll tell you what to do as we go along.'

At least the patient was asleep and didn't realise what was happening. All went well anyway and baby Sian was born fit and healthy, despite my lack of surgical skills.

The more I worked with him, the more I came to respect Lionel's expertise. I'll never forget the day a lady called Katie was sent to the antenatal clinic to see him. She was planning a home birth, but her baby was in a breech or feet-first position and she and her midwife agreed that a doctor's opinion should be sought. It can be a risk to give birth at home to a breech baby, but Katie was adamant that she did not want to go into hospital. Her mother had recently died at the hospital and she was still very upset. Lionel listened to her story and was sympathetic about her bereavement. Then he examined her and told her to go home and plan a home birth. She anxiously asked him about the baby's position. 'Oh, I've turned the baby round while we've been talking,' he explained. She hadn't felt a thing!

Turning breech babies is no longer the common procedure it once was. It can be dangerous if not done by a very skilled operator and is usually carried out on the labour ward now, in case complications arise and an emergency caesarean is needed. Lionel had many years of experience and was able to do it quickly and safely in the clinic. He completely understood that going into the hospital where her mother had died would traumatise Katie, who went on to have a wonderful home birth and was very grateful for Lionel's help.

The antenatal and postnatal wards were known as Nightingale wards and laid out in a very traditional way. The beds were in two long rows and the midwives' table was in the middle of the ward. The beds had curtains for privacy, but these were rarely used, which meant that the midwives could chat to all the women and they could chat to each other. A jolly midwife called Jan used to push herself round the ward in a wheelchair just for fun; she would cheer up all the mums who had 'the blues'. She often had us all in fits of laughter . . . I might have said 'she had us in stitches', but that wouldn't be appropriate! As well as being a natural entertainer, Jan was very competent and caring. They say laughter is the best medicine and it certainly seemed to do the mothers good. I suspect that her behaviour would not be tolerated these days.

Some of the midwives at my new hospital were real characters. Alison, whom I met on my first day, absolutely terrified me! She was tall and had a commanding presence (her husband called her bossy) but she was immense fun to work with. She was also very good at putting doctors in their place if necessary – and it *was* necessary every now and then. Her self-assurance and confidence were inspiring and I wished I could be like her.

I was sorry when she left to take up a rather prestigious

nursing post, but it wasn't too long before I saw her again, this time as a patient. She had given birth to her first baby and was in the postnatal ward suffering from very painful stitches. I gently removed them for her and she was thrilled that she was able to walk properly again. I saw her then as a mother, rather than a high-powered professional, and we became firm friends. I felt very privileged when she asked me to deliver her second baby.

Alison enjoys telling people about the experience. 'Agnes was so bossy when I was in labour and she took the gas and air away from me when I still needed it.' I'm not sure I was all that bossy; I think she just wasn't used to having someone else in charge!

Another friend, Anne, initially appeared to be the opposite of Alison. She was very petite, but I soon discovered that what she lacked in height, she made up for in temperament and spirit. I admired the way she always spoke her mind; she wasn't half as bothered as I was about being polite and diplomatic. Anne's character had been shaped by her childhood. She had lived in a children's home until she was seven and her birth mother died before she managed to trace her. It was very sad, especially as her adoptive mother never showed her any love or affection. She was sent to boarding school, which made her very independent and self-assured, and she always argued for what she believed in – a trait we shared.

Once, she was assisting a consultant with the delivery of a private patient's baby. The midwives were obliged to help out with private cases, even though they received no extra pay for doing so, something many of them found unfair and unethical, because the consultants charged a lot of money for their services. 'Give me the obstetric forceps, please,' the consultant barked at Anne. 'It looks like I need to get this baby delivered now.'

'No, you don't need them!' Anne said bravely, refusing to hand them over. 'She doesn't need forceps; she can push the baby out herself.' Which the woman promptly did.

The consultant was shocked. She wasn't used to being told what to do, especially by a five-foot-nothing midwife. 'Do you speak to your husband that way?' she asked Anne later.

'Yes, I do, and he's six foot four!' Anne retorted. Her suspicion was that the consultant had only been keen to employ the use of instruments in order to charge a bigger fee for the delivery. Meanwhile Anne was acting in the woman's best interests, as a midwife must always do. How I admired her bravado!

Despite Anne's difficult childhood, she made a very happy and lasting marriage and produced three children, who are a joy and a credit to her. It was Anne in whom I confided when I fell in love again, after being on my own for eight years. How did it happen? Well, it's quite a strange story, or so some of my friends seemed to think.

7

Love Second Time Around

I wasn't looking for love. A little romance, maybe, but a long-term partner was the last thing on my mind. I was busy, happy, fulfilled in my job and I had my children already. But as is often the way, when I was least expecting it, suddenly, there it was. It started when I took my children to Tenerife for a holiday. The boys were nine and ten at the time and it was the first time I'd taken them abroad, as we had not been able to afford such luxuries in the past. I was supposed to be taking a friend with me, but she pulled out at the last minute, because her boyfriend, Mohammed, didn't want her to go on holiday with a divorcée. Once there, I had my eye on the tour guide, who was quite handsome, but I wasn't interested in anybody else at all.

In the evenings at our hotel, the boys would go to bed and I'd go to the bar with a couple I'd met. They came from near where I lived; they were really nice and I got on well with them. Another holidaymaker, Derek, also tagged along; he was on his own as well, because his friend had also let him down at the last minute. So the four of us would sit at the bar and chat or walk to the town; we clicked as a group.

At the airport on the way home, I gave the couple my

address. Derek was sitting there and I thought I'd better give it to him as well, otherwise it would look rude. Still, I never expected to see him again. Nothing had happened. We'd just got on well.

A few weeks later, out of the blue, Derek wrote to say that he was working in the area and could we meet up? Well, I was rehearsing in the school pantomime the night we arranged to meet. I was playing Robin Hood, wearing a pair of shorts! It was really embarrassing. Derek came along to the rehearsal; that was his first date with me. The next time we saw each other, he came for the weekend and one thing led to another. We ended up on the sofa . . .

I think he might have had the idea all along, although he would never admit it. All the while, I was oblivious. But I just felt so easy in his company and the more I got to know him, the more I liked him. We only spent a few weekends together – twelve days, to be precise – before I suddenly thought, 'He's the one!' Obviously, between times we wrote to each other and talked on the phone. It was all happening so fast, and I was elated, but also shocked. I had been on my own for such a long time, so I was very independent. But I wasn't a naive young girl anymore, I had enough experience of life to know that this was something special, so I decided to just go with it, even though I hadn't been looking for a partner.

The fact that he was so much younger than me was unusual as well. He was twenty-two and I was thirty, divorced with two children. His parents were very apprehensive. I sympathised, because I would have felt the same if it had been my son. 'Don't tell them about me until I've met them,' I said to him. 'Give me a chance to meet them first.' It really helped, because they got to know me a bit as a person, rather than as A Single Mother – a very daunting-sounding label.

Derek had already got to know my boys a little on holiday, but that had been as an acquaintance. Now I was anxious about the impact this new relationship would have on my children. But we took things gently and everyone got on fine.

Derek and I got married six months after we first met, which is probably not most people's idea of a recipe for a lasting union! Anne, for instance, had known her husband Alan for several years before they even got engaged – and they'd had a long engagement before getting married. She thought I was being very hasty hitching myself to a man who was eight years my junior and lived at home with his parents. Her disapproval of my impending nuptials was considerable. 'I'll give it six months,' she said in her usual forthright way whenever we talked about it.

On the other hand, my mother completely supported me in my decision. 'If you know he's the one, then go ahead and marry him and don't listen to anyone else,' she said simply.

I'm pleased to say that my dear outspoken friend was wrong and my beloved husband and I are still together after thirty years. Some people say we look the same age now, despite the eight-year difference, as over the years being with me has robbed him of his figure, his looks, his hair and his salary . . . all of which has aged him!

Despite her initial cynicism about my second marriage,

Anne and I continued to be great friends, and we were also very close to a wonderful midwife called Stella. Just as her name suggests, Stella was a star. With her golden, pixie-cropped hair and sunshine smile, she was a beautiful girl who could easily have been a model. Her whole face lit up when she smiled and, unlike some good-looking people, she wasn't in the least bit vain.

She genuinely loved helping people. An experienced nurse and midwife, she also had many other talents: she was an excellent dressmaker and cook and, to my surprise, a DIY wizard. I thought wiring a plug was quite an achievement, but Stella could retile a roof or floor and fit kitchen cupboards with ease!

Stella's husband, Malcolm, was a kind and funny man, a respected art teacher who always longed to have his own pottery. After they decided to move to the Isle of Wight to start their own business, they renovated a property there and eventually ran a successful pottery and bistro.

However, disaster was waiting to strike, as it randomly does. Malcolm was diagnosed with facial cancer and began a gruelling period of surgery and chemotherapy. Even though he lost an eye and part of his palate, he bravely fought the illness for the next five years. During this period, Stella was desperate to have a child, but Malcolm became infertile because of the cancer treatment. They decided to seek help from a specialist in London and agreed to try artificial insemination with donor sperm. Happily, the treatment succeeded and they were delighted when she gave birth to a son.

Unfortunately, Stella suffered from severe postnatal

depression and never seemed to fully recover. From time to time we would all meet up when she came over to the mainland, but it was clear that she was not the happy-go-lucky girl she used to be, especially when she told us about the strange thoughts and feelings she was experiencing. We were so worried that we contacted her health visitor on the island to voice our concern.

Although Malcolm continued to battle cancer, Stella decided to have another child. She had artificial insemination by donor again and this time conceived twins, giving birth in the hospital where she had worked as a midwife while she and Malcolm were setting up their pottery business. Just after the babies' birth, while she was resting in bed, she claimed to be bleeding very heavily. She was concerned that the midwives did not take her worries seriously. So she struggled out of bed, staggered to the public telephone outside the ward and rang the consultant obstetrician on call.

'If you don't come and see me, I'm going to die of a haemorrhage!' she warned him.

When she related this story to us, we were unsure whether her anxiety was justified or if it was an indicator of her increasingly fragile state of mind. It was so hard to know, but we suspected that something was very wrong.

Eventually the pottery and bistro had to close down because of Malcolm's illness and the couple moved to Northumberland. Stella cared for Malcolm as well as she could, but this took its toll on her and she was forced to allow the children to be cared for by foster parents for several days a week.

After five years of fighting his illness, sadly Malcolm died. By now, Stella's heart and spirit were broken and her mental state declined still further. One day, when she was alone at home, she took a fatal overdose. Her death left us all shocked and bewildered. How could this tragedy have happened to such a beautiful star?

One thing is for certain, those of us who knew Stella will always remember her with love and admiration. Her sad story made us all very aware of the damage that post-natal depression can cause. Back then, we knew so much less about it than we do now – and, thankfully, new treatments are beginning to show results in this area. How tragic that developments in this field came too late to help our wonderful Stella. We can only hope that her children will find the peace and happiness that they surely deserve.

I came across an alarming case of postnatal depression at my local hospital. It concerned a lady named Michelle, who had a severe form of the illness called puerperal psychosis. It is so serious that the woman completely loses touch with reality and does not even realise she's ill. When I met Michelle, she had given birth to her first child five days previously. A pretty girl with long dark hair, she was twenty-six and worked as a beauty consultant. In the days after the birth, she complained of being unable to sleep and her behaviour became increasingly strange. By chance, one of the nursing auxiliaries saw her leave the ward with her baby in her arms and climb a flight of stairs leading to an unused nursery on the floor above. Instinct told the nurse to follow and she entered the nursery to find Michelle climbing up on to the window ledge.

'I was just about to throw the baby out of the window,' she confessed later.

The psychiatrist who counselled Michelle could not find any reason for her action and believed it to be due to severe hormonal instability. Certainly, her circumstances appeared not to be a factor: she and her husband had a happy married life, were buying their first house and both had good jobs. Happily, after spending several months in a special mother and baby psychiatric unit and being treated with medication, she was fit and well and back to her normal self.

Postnatal depression strikes indiscriminately and, although recognised as an illness by the medical profession, is still not completely understood. It occurs in about one in seven to one in ten women. Often medication or hormone therapy is used but some doctors believe that counselling is the best treatment. Puerperal psychosis is much less common and affects about one in five hundred women. Neither illness should be confused with the 'baby blues', which is a normal, transient condition that affects up to two-thirds of new mothers. The baby blues is a feeling of emotional instability and low mood that occurs because of hormone changes a few days after the birth. One minute a woman can be sobbing and the next minute she might be cracking up with laughter. Partners are usually advised to tread very carefully during this time, as saying something quite innocent, or arriving to visit a few minutes late, can cause an unprecedented outburst of tears from a new mum. But the 'baby blues' only lasts a day or two before things settle down again. Having worked in the field all my life, I know how vital it is that mothers get the postnatal care they need, to avoid more tragedies like Stella's.

Night duty was an essential part of our working lives at the hospital. It could be a really busy shift or a quiet one with a chance to catch up on your knitting. One particular evening, a jolly midwife called Diane decided to ring a colleague, Joyce, to ask her to change a shift the next day. To obtain an outside telephone line it was necessary to dial nine first. However, Diane forgot to do this and unfortunately the first three digits of Joyce's phone number were the same as the fire emergency number in the hospital. Pandemonium ensued! The alarm bell rang in the fire station and within a few minutes the sirens of two fire engines could be heard in the distance. A member of staff from each ward hurried to a central meeting point to find out where the fire was and whether it was necessary to evacuate their patients. I was the person who went from our department. I was shocked to learn the fire was somewhere in the maternity unit. While rushing back from the meeting point, I met two gorgeous firemen bounding up the stairs to the labour ward.

'Where's the fire, love?' they asked, panting furiously.

Diane's face was a picture of horror as she realised what she'd done. Fortunately, the firemen were magnanimous about the situation and we all parted friends. Diane, however, spent the night worrying that she would have to foot the bill for a call-out to a false alarm. As it happened, she wasn't held responsible, but she wrote a letter of apology to the hospital administrator just in case.

We came to expect the unexpected on night duty. One evening at dusk, I happened to be working with a medical student called Steve, because as well as training student midwives we sometimes mentored medical students from one of the London teaching hospitals. Suddenly there was a power cut – and astonishingly the hospital's emergency generator also broke down. We were left in almost complete darkness. As luck would have it, at that very moment a woman arrived in the department with her husband. She was in the last stages of labour and although I couldn't see her very well, I could tell by her noisy breathing that I had to get her into a delivery room quickly. Recalling where the only torch in the ward was, I groped my way over to find it. Steve held it expertly and shortly afterwards the woman gave birth to a lovely baby boy, whom I managed to catch easily in the twilight.

It was probably much nicer for the baby to be born into a peaceful, dimly lit environment than the usual noisy, fluorescent lit one. Soon afterwards, the power was restored and everyone was most surprised to see Steve and me emerging from the room with a baby. They had been so busy panicking and running around that they hadn't noticed the couple coming in.

Steve was a rare student. He had so much compassion and common sense. He looked after one woman in labour so well that a paediatrician who was asked to attend the birth mistook him for the woman's husband! He was funny and a little bit cheeky and all the staff loved him.

When there was a farewell party for Adela, one of the doctors, he transformed himself into her lookalike by putting on a dress, applying full make-up and sporting an enormous plait just like the one she always wore. He then read a very irreverent poem he had made up about her, to hoots of laughter from all her colleagues.

The fun times were essential in counteracting the serious times. Just before I started working at the hospital, a woman called Grace had died in childbirth. This was an extremely rare and shocking experience which affected all the staff very badly. Miss Griffiths described what had happened, in order to warn me of the danger of preeclampsia, a condition peculiar to pregnancy.

Grace, who was expecting her second child, had been diagnosed with pre-eclampsia a couple of weeks before she was due. One of the symptoms is high blood pressure, which can be dangerous for both mother and baby. During the labour, Grace's blood pressure had risen alarmingly and Joan, her midwife, had called the doctor to attend.

But it was the middle of the night and the doctor was unwilling to come to the ward. He instructed that Grace be given an injection of pethidine, which would hopefully lower her blood pressure and ease her pain. However, her blood pressure continued to rise and Joan anxiously telephoned the doctor again. He reluctantly agreed to attend. Grace then suffered a fit and lost consciousness, at which point Joan called for urgent assistance and a resuscitation team arrived. A consultant obstetrician performed an emergency caesarean section and baby Cathy was safely delivered. Grace, though, was transferred to the intensive care unit but never regained consciousness. She died a week later.

Grace's husband Neil was distraught. When he discovered the facts of what had happened that night, he became angry at what he believed had been the needless loss of his wife. He took his case to court and six years later was awarded a few thousand pounds' compensation. The doctor was criticised for not attending sooner, but no action could be taken because he had left the country by that time. Although the pitiful compensation awarded was certainly not enough to provide a substitute mother for Cathy, she grew up to be a lovely girl and a credit to her father. Her mother would have been so proud of her. Some years later, Neil remarried and had more children, but he told me that each time his wife gave birth he was reminded of the nightmare of Grace's death. Indeed, how could he not be?

One of the reasons I found my job so challenging was that I never knew what was in store when I arrived at the hospital each day. Soon after I started, a very unusual and distressing birth took place. The baby's head and shoulders were delivered, but then the baby became completely stuck. The doctor and midwife were puzzled. What could the problem be? They decided that a cyst on the baby's back might be causing the problem, so a decision was made to operate.

Since the operating theatre was on the floor below and at the end of a long corridor, the poor baby had to be assisted to breathe on the journey. Meanwhile, the mother suffered the trauma of being pushed on a trolley with her baby half in and half out. In the theatre, her abdomen was opened and the cyst drained before the rest of the baby was delivered. Miraculously, the baby survived. It had an unusual condition, but grew up to be healthy and normal. I'm glad to say that the introduction of ultrasound scanning has meant such problems are very rarely left undetected these days.

Before scanning became so routine, it was up to the midwife or doctor to detect the presence of twins. The doctors used to deliver them; it wasn't left to the midwives, so I had very little experience with them. If one twin is breech, they usually offer a caesarean now, but having twins wasn't considered such a risk then as is it now. One of my colleagues was expecting twins and they were both head first, so another colleague delivered the first one and when the doctor came to check that the second one was in the right place, he delivered the second one.

My husband is a twin and his mother told me that there were several hours between the birth of the first and the second. In those days it was quite common to have a long gap between twin births, but nowadays it's minutes: they wouldn't let them sit in there for hours. There's always a risk that, after the first is born, the second twin might turn and lie horizontally; it's a worry, because this could rupture the uterus. The doctors are so scared of this possibility that they often advise a caesarean. Still, I've worked with a midwife who delivers twins all the time, head first and breech. She's happy doing it, and has never had a problem, so I don't think they should necessarily be delivered by caesarean section.

Because of the lack of scanning, at least once or twice a year twins were born when only one baby was expected. This was a shock for the parents, albeit a pleasant one. I remember one father joyfully heading off to make a telephone call to his family to tell them about the arrival of his son, only to be given a huge surprise when he returned to the delivery room.

'Well, dear, you're a lucky man; you've now got two sons!' the midwife told him jovially.

He passed out on the spot! But once over their initial shock, both parents were very happy and pleased with themselves. Childbirth is always a life-changing event, but sometimes in surprising ways.

8

Motherhood Again
1981

About a year after I began working at my local hospital, my husband and I decided to have a baby. My children were eleven and twelve years old and, although I was only thirty, I didn't want the age gap between them and the new baby to be any wider.

I became pregnant straight away, but how different it was this time. I was terrified! When I had my boys, I knew nothing about having babies and ignorance was definitely bliss. This time I knew too much and I worried about everything. I fretted about things most women have never heard of and I kept my husband Derek awake at night telling him scary birth stories!

Things went from bad to worse. I had chosen to have this baby at home like my other two children, but no-one appeared willing to support my decision. Maternity services had changed so much over the previous eleven years that home births had gradually been phased out. The community midwife attached to the surgery was never available for me to talk to, and she would not have gone against the doctor's advice anyway. Like many doctors, my GP was scared of home births. It's understandable when you consider that they probably never get to see one during their training. They only have to deliver a few babies before they qualify as doctors, unlike midwives, who must deliver forty. What's more, when they work in a maternity department, they are only called to the labour ward if there are difficulties with a birth. So it follows that they see birth as a potentially dangerous situation and, worse, these days as a possible cause of litigation. I also sensed that my GP was nervous of me, because he felt I knew more about pregnancy than he did. This was probably true, even though I had not been a midwife very long, about three years.

He decided at a routine check-up early on that I must be expecting twins, because I was quite large. He asked me to feel my own tummy, but this was quite difficult from my position lying on the couch! Hearing that my husband is a twin reinforced his belief and he packed me off to see the consultant obstetrician at the hospital where I worked.

This experience made me begin to question in earnest the way women were dealt with during their pregnancies. It seemed to me that things were done in a certain way for no good reason other than that they were routine practice. For example, why did women have to strip off for their first booking appointment? As I sat in the corridor of the antenatal clinic waiting for the consultant obstetrician to arrive, wearing an old dressing gown that had been worn by many other women, I felt a loss of dignity and a loss of control. I dearly hoped the gown had been laundered.

Was this a ploy to show the medical profession's power over its patients? I came to believe that it was. I hated the practice even more when I later worked with a seedy consultant who would almost be licking his lips with glee as he entered the consulting room. He used to examine the women's breasts and pronounce them able to breastfeed, which was all totally unnecessary. Sometimes he did a vaginal examination, for no real reason. I felt he was a dirty old man, but since stripping for the booking appointment was policy across the country, there wasn't anything I could do or say about it. It's not policy anymore, because it was realised that there's no value whatsoever in a consultant seeing a normal healthy pregnant woman for that first appointment. It's much better to see a midwife. But in those days you had to sit there naked and vulnerable.

I wasn't a patient. I wasn't ill. I was pregnant. I was an intelligent, professional woman, for heaven's sake, so why was I allowing this to happen to me? And if I – a midwife – couldn't object, then how could other women be expected to do so?

At least my consultant was a lady, thank goodness! When she scanned me with the portable machine in the clinic, she found only one baby. I must admit I would have been happy to have twins. But my GP had apparently been right that there was something unusual about this pregnancy.

'You have a fibroid in the uterus, I'm afraid,' she told me. 'That means you must have a hospital birth, in case you haemorrhage after the delivery.'

I was terribly disappointed not to be able to have a home birth, but at the time I felt that it was a good thing that I had been seen by the doctor – despite my feeling that it could have been handled better. Fibroids are benign growths that can cause problems such as pain, heavy periods and even infertility for some women. I had never had any symptoms at all, but this discovery meant I really did have something to worry about now! My GP heaved a sigh of relief that I was off his hands; and so the nightmare of being on the other side continued.

I saw the consultant for every check-up after that. Maybe she did it as a professional courtesy, but seeing her scared me. Although she was charming, she sometimes thought out loud and made me worry unnecessarily. Before this experience, I think I may have dismissed some women's anxieties without really understanding them. In future, I knew I would have much more empathy. It made me understand, too, that it is easy to interpret what is said very differently from how it is meant, just because warnings about pre-eclampsia, gestational diabetes and premature birth can sound quite terrifying if you don't get a sense of the statistics and likelihood of them happening.

I felt very vulnerable, especially when the consultant examined me internally, which she did frequently, with that instrument of female torture known as a speculum. It is a device which is inserted into the vagina and has two small wings which can be screwed open in order to hold the vagina in a position so that the cervix is visible. One day, as she screwed it open, it pinched a bit of my skin! Oh, the pain . . . it made my eyes water . . . but I didn't say anything. I just gritted my teeth until it was over! I have no idea what she was looking for, or whether she ever found it, as she never told me and I was too fearful to ask.

I liked the consultant and respected her, but it seemed strange to be her patient after having worked with her. I found it intimidating, because I was a bit scared of her. She was quite an imposing woman who had no children because she had married late in life after concentrating on her career. She was good at her job, but I felt she did not really understand the emotional aspects of childbirth. She did write me a nice reference, though, when I was applying for a promotion to a higher grade. But that wasn't much consolation when I was being examined on her consulting bed, wondering what on earth was going on.

Eventually, when I was five days past my due date, she made a decision. 'I think it would be for the best if we induced this baby.' I wasn't sure this was necessary, but felt completely unable to argue.

When I was admitted to hospital, it was hard to know whether I should behave like a patient or a midwife. Should I have coffee in the office with my friends, or should I join the other women in the ward? The upshot of this conundrum is that I have always treated pregnant medical professionals just like everybody else, because I know now we are all the same. It doesn't matter how much you know, you still need the same reassurance, respect and kindness as the next woman.

Another thing I learned was that enemas are horrendous! They were given routinely at that time, but why? Tradition? I swore never to inflict an enema on anyone again without a very good reason. I wasn't surprised when I later read that research had proved there was no discernible benefit to giving enemas before labour.

My lovely husband wanted to be as supportive as possible, but he had no idea what to do for me during labour because I didn't let him attend any antenatal classes. This was one of those impulsive decisions that you regret afterwards. I think I thought it would be boring for both of us to have to sit there with him listening to somebody teaching me what I taught other people. I thought I could probably tell Derek what he needed to know, but actually it is quite different teaching your husband about your own baby to teaching a bunch of strangers, and somehow I never got round to it, thinking that I was the one who needed to know everything. I shot myself in the foot there, didn't I? Still, he enjoyed watching Wimbledon on television while I got on with coping with the contractions!

In my case, induction was not a good idea. My previous labours had been unusually quick; a first labour usually lasts twelve to sixteen hours and mine had lasted three. The second took only two hours. To make matters worse, at this third labour, I was given a drug of a larger dose than necessary because the smaller dose could not be found in the drug fridge! This caused me to have massive contractions for twenty minutes. Janet, the midwife looking after me, later told me that she had feared my uterus would rupture. Baby Tom was born so quickly that he was shocked and had to be whisked away to be resuscitated in another room. This memory haunts me still. What happened to him when I wasn't there? How long was it before he breathed?

Eventually, he was returned to us and we were left alone with him, entranced, excited and euphoric. Thinking about it later, it occurred to me that the birth of this little person linked each of us together in our new family. I could not have been happier. Once again I was a proud mum and I felt ecstatic.

The feelings of joy and wonder and achievement were the same as with my other two boys, but in one crucial way this hospital birth was very different. I spent that night in a room on my own; my baby lay in the nursery down the corridor, as was the usual practice. My husband went home to the other children. Without my baby next to me, I felt as if part of my body had been amputated. We should all have been together at such a crucial time in our lives. And during our short stay in hospital, Tom caught an infection from another baby and had to be treated with antibiotics. I worried about the effect this would have on his brand new immune system, but I had no choice but to give them to him. Since I had not haemorrhaged, and indeed at a later check-up after the birth the mysterious fibroid had disappeared, I wondered whether I had really needed to give birth in hospital at all.

These events made me seriously question the wisdom of the Government's drive towards hospital birth for all. I felt that for many women home birth would be a much better experience. As for women with complications, in my opinion their partners and children should be able to stay with them in family-sized rooms. But that dream is probably still a long way off for the NHS hospitals in this country, although I know there are a couple of places where it happens.

To try to exorcise the bad memories of this birth experience, I decided to write a short article for a well-known baby magazine. The theme of the piece was what happens

when midwives themselves have babies. I got the idea
from a woman who had attended antenatal classes I had
taught. She was a freelance journalist and she remarked
one day that I must have a rich supply of stories to tell
about childbirth. This prompted me to tell my own story
and, despite it being my first foray into the world of writing, it was accepted for publication and I earned fifty
pounds. This was a great deal of money for me in 1981
and writing about my dissatisfaction helped me to come
to terms with it.

However, when I arrived at work a few days after the
magazine had been published, there was a shock awaiting
me. A copy of my article was pinned up on the wall and it
was entitled 'SHOULD MIDWIVES BE MOTHERS?' I
had tried to express, perhaps clumsily, that we cannot fully
know what effect our actions have on a woman unless we
have been on the receiving end ourselves, so we should
always be mindful of their feelings. But this had been
misinterpreted by some people who thought I was suggesting that all midwives should be mothers themselves. This
upset those colleagues who had not yet had a baby and in
particular the one or two who had been unable to conceive.
Of course I didn't mean to hurt anyone. Anyway, I had
known some wonderful midwives who didn't have their
own children, so I would never have suggested that you
couldn't do a good job if you were childless.

But sadly the damage was done. A piece of paper had
been pinned underneath the article for comments and
people had vented their feelings. In addition, a group of
my colleagues were sitting in a room waiting for me to

arrive for my shift, ready to harangue me. It felt like a scene from the Spanish Inquisition!

I was terribly upset. I felt I had suffered a traumatic birth but I wasn't blaming any one person; I was saying that the system was at fault. I have always genuinely wanted the best care for women and that's why I have always been prepared to question why things are done the way they are.

It took me a long while to get over the incident and I had to apologise publicly to everyone, but thank goodness I decided not to resign, even though I felt like it at the time. Since then, of course, things have changed a lot, so perhaps I was just ahead of my time.

I subsequently had my first daughter, Lucy, a gorgeous baby who made our family complete. Again, I wanted to give birth at home, but was persuaded not to. I didn't feel strong enough to argue against the doctor's advice. I think this happens to women a lot when they are pregnant. They are vulnerable and scared, and sometimes they are simply too tired to resist an overbearing doctor. Even I, with all my experience, felt unable to stand up for what I wanted and believed in. I find this incredible now, but I think perhaps I had been spooked by the experience with the mystery fibroid. In any case, I complied.

I started getting labour contractions in the middle of the night and my husband awoke to a vision of me performing contortions as I tried to examine myself internally to check if my cervix was dilating.

'What on earth are you doing?' he asked, looking perplexed.

'It's ridiculous, I know!' I said. 'But I don't want to be sent home for going in too early.'

Actually, I didn't manage to find my cervix, but I went to hospital anyway. This time things were better and a good friend of mine, Barbara, delivered my baby. When I started to tell her what to do, she wisely told me to shut up and let her get on with it!

When the paediatrician came to examine Lucy the next morning, prior to us going home, she started choking. I wasn't terribly worried because new babies often have mucus in their throats and I just expected the doctor to deal with it. However, it was obvious he didn't know what to do, so I rang the bell for a midwife who came and sorted Lucy out quickly and efficiently. The poor doctor was embarrassed, but he had an excuse, as it was his first day in the maternity department. Later he became a GP and we met again when I was a community midwife.

'Agnes! I remember that day we first met,' he said. 'I didn't know one end of a baby from the other and it really scared me.' He is a superb doctor and I admired him for admitting his shortcomings, a rare quality in the medical profession. He is justly very popular with his patients.

I was very lucky to be in a job where I could work part-time, and when Lucy was a few months old I returned to work for a few hours a week. They say pregnant women and new mothers lose their brain power and I think this is true. Luckily, I was sent to the antenatal clinic, where I couldn't do much damage, although sometimes people would speak to me and I would turn round and totally forget what they had said.

Still, I enjoyed going back to work, being a midwife again and also being myself for a few hours and not just 'Mum'. I couldn't have done it without my mother's help though. She cheerfully volunteered to look after all the children, whenever necessary. She was so proud of me that she would have done anything to help me continue with the career that she knew I loved. When she died of leukaemia at the age of seventy in 1988, it was the saddest day of my life. Her loss blotted out everything else for a while. It had been an agonising few months in the run-up to her death and the whole family was exhausted and numb with sadness. I felt I had to support my children, who were having to learn to cope with bereavement, but I could hardly function myself.

My mother was the most important person to me and had the biggest influence on me. She supported me in whatever I did and never judged or criticised me. She loved all her children and grandchildren equally and they were all she lived for. I wish my children had been able to have more time with her. She had a difficult life because of my father's alcoholism, but protected her children from it as much as she could, and managed to remain cheerful despite her own health problems. She struggled to have a proper social life, because she was very hard of hearing and hearing aids were not as technically advanced as they are now. She was brave and uncomplaining, even when suffering from the effects of the leukaemia and was still concerned more for other people than herself.

Having lived through the war years, like many of her contemporaries she was very thrifty and, unknown to us children, she saved enough to give us each a nice nest egg when she died. This was more important to her than spending money on herself. But best of all, we laughed a lot together; she had a wonderful sense of humour.

I was already feeling some very complex emotions and was tired and low when I lost her. My father had died of pneumonia and alcoholism three months before she died. He was a very clever man and in his own way he loved his family; he had many good qualities and his addiction was a cruel illness. When he died, I naively thought it would be a relief for my mother, after all the years of worry. But she loved him despite everything and she was broken-hearted at his death, perhaps grieving for the husband she never had.

Even now, over twenty years after her death, I can feel tears coming into my eyes when I write about her. She was such a special person that everybody loved her fiercely. I can only wish for the same relationship with my own children.

With my mother no longer around to babysit for me, I worried that I would not be able to continue working. Our new midwife manager, Mrs Murnaghan – or Mrs M, as she was fondly known – was very sympathetic when I explained my situation.

'It's all right, love,' she reassured me. 'You can simply work when your husband's around to look after the children. Let me know which hours and days you can do and I'll sort out the duty rota.' This was great news and definitely the most advantageous way to treat your staff. Mrs

M knew that when my circumstances changed, I would work more hours – and because of her sympathetic and flexible approach, I always helped her out when she needed me. Just like Miss Griffiths, she valued all her staff and was rewarded by having an extremely loyal team.

I loved working in the antenatal clinic and getting to know the mums-to-be, and sometimes their partners and other children. My work was a wonderful distraction from the pain of losing Mum, as it simply isn't possible to mope when you have a busy clinic to run. The women's first visit was usually for a booking appointment, when their medical history was taken. Occasionally a woman attended who already had six or more children and it took ages to get all the information about the pregnancies and birth dates down on paper, as inevitably she would forget things. Often women did not realise the importance of some events and would not mention them. Of course it was even more difficult if their first language wasn't English!

I made sure that I was sensitive to the women's feelings and fears. I never forgot what I had learned in the gynaecology ward when I was training, when I realised what a terrible experience having a miscarriage can be. When you're taking a history from someone when they're pregnant, you always ask, 'Have you had any pregnancies before?'

If they said, 'Yes, I had a miscarriage last year,' I made sure to pause and say, 'Really sorry to hear that. How did you cope?' before going on to ask how many weeks pregnant they had been and all the other necessary medical information. I was aware that most people don't get the chance to talk about their miscarriage, and often they have to cope with it on their own.

Sometimes women came to the clinic for a check-up during their pregnancy, although most went to their GP's surgery to see their allocated midwife. Some women came to see the obstetricians if they had complications with their pregnancy, or medical conditions such as diabetes. In 1969, when I had my first baby, there were no screening tests available to check that your baby was going to be healthy. Now parents can choose to have a test to find out how likely they are to have a baby with either Down's syndrome or spina bifida. These tests are called screening tests, because they only give a risk factor. If the risk factor shows there is a possible problem, the parents can go on to have further tests that will provide a definite diagnosis.

These are difficult decisions for some people to make: firstly whether to have the test in the first place and secondly what to do about the result. Some parents feel they cannot cope with a disabled child and choose to have a termination. Others do not want to end the pregnancy either way, but want to know whether their child will be affected, so they can prepare themselves. Some people simply say that they will love and accept the baby they are given and choose not to have the tests at all.

Many people I've talked to at the beginning of pregnancy have no idea that they have these test options; neither has the possibility that there might be something wrong with their baby entered their heads. When I mention screening to them, often they don't know what to do, and I've been asked my opinion countless times. I always explain that I am happy to give all the information, but that the decision must be theirs and I will support them in whatever they choose to do.

I can't deny that it sometimes used to make me feel uncomfortable when people declared outright that they wouldn't want a baby with any problems at all. This is because when I was born I was thought to be blind. It must have been dreadful for my mother, because nobody talked to her or gave her an explanation. They just said, 'Your baby's probably going to be blind. It would be best to put her in a home, forget about her and try again.'

It seems incredible these days to think that someone would say such a thing, but it was the 1940s. I can't imagine how my mother must have felt, especially as she wouldn't have dreamt of putting me in a home. What's more, only one of my eyes was affected, not both of them; how could they make that mistake? I actually have some sight in the bad eye, not enough to read, but probably enough to stop me falling over the chairs. My consultant thinks that because I've had the problem from birth, I probably turn my head to see more than other people.

My mother never told me the story; I only found it out after she had died and my aunt recalled the day I was born, when my mother had phoned her from the hospital in tears. She said my mother was heartbroken – not for herself, but for me and what life would hold for me. Of course, although it has caused me some difficulties, I've lived a full, active life and pursued a challenging career, so the doctors were completely mistaken. And one day when we were discussing my sight problem, my mother told me that I had been a joy to her, which made me realise that it doesn't matter if your child is different, you love them anyway.

So sometimes when parents are adamant about not having a baby who is anything but healthy and normal, it does make me want to question them about where to draw the line when it comes to terminating babies who are not perfect. But of course I don't ever voice my feelings.

I also have an inherited hearing problem, so when people bring up worries about having a child with health complications, I used to say, 'Look at me. I'm really deaf, with funny eyes, and I've still got degrees and everything!' I used my example to make people feel better, if I could.

One couple found out that their baby had Down's syndrome and a major heart defect at thirty-six weeks of pregnancy. The mother had been sent for a scan because the midwife thought there was extra fluid in the uterus, a condition which can indicate that there is a problem with the baby. The scan had picked up a heart defect common to children with Down's syndrome and so the mother had further tests, which confirmed the doctors' suspicions. I was standing in for the couple's midwife that day and the father rang me in a very distraught state while they were awaiting the results. When I arrived at their house, they had just been telephoned and told the news. The mother was wailing and the father was sobbing and I didn't know how to comfort or console them. The father was angry that the condition had not been discovered before, especially as the mother had had a screening test at the beginning of the pregnancy and it had not shown anything abnormal. Parents are counselled before the test that it is not a hundred per cent accurate, so there is no legal redress.

I arranged for the couple to have counselling and to discuss their options with experts. They were told that it was difficult to know how long the baby would live after birth because of its heart condition. Eventually, after the shedding of many tears, they decided to terminate the pregnancy. This is not a decision taken lightly at this stage of pregnancy, with just four weeks to go until the due date. It involved the baby being given an injection via the uterus that would end its life. The mother then had to go home and come back to the hospital later for labour to be induced. Whether one agrees with termination or not, it must have been a truly dreadful thing to experience. The parents told me later that some of the midwives had treated them less than kindly, which I think is unacceptable. We do not have the right to judge other people's decisions and beliefs; our job is simply to give support.

I saw a lot of judging going on within hospital walls: of unmarried women earlier on in my career and then of young girls who came in with pierced eyebrows and noses. You can't help being judgemental; I think it's human nature. We all make assumptions merely by looking at somebody. But as a professional, you must try not to treat them any differently; you don't have to act as if you're judging them. You can perhaps go back to the office and say, 'Did you see that woman?' but you don't have to reveal what you're thinking when you're with them.

I found it pretty easy to put my opinions to one side. Although I was probably making judgements internally, I always tried not to show it. I was careful because I had been judged myself when I was a nineteen-year-old mother and it hadn't been a pleasant experience. Nobody knew how I was going to end up, so they had no right to judge me. That's why I would always hesitate to judge other people.

Some problems that crop up at an antenatal clinic appointment are impossible to deal with in the fifteen-minute slot allotted. For instance, a caesarean section will be advised for most women who have a baby in an awkward position at thirty-six weeks of pregnancy, as it is thought to be safer for the baby. They may be disappointed by this, but I used to assure them that it can be a positive experience.

'Well, at least you know when the birthday will be,' I'd tell them, 'and you will be able to get everything organised beforehand. That must be an advantage!'

Understandably, they want to talk through the implications of the operation and that can take quite a bit of time. Some women understand and don't mind if they are kept waiting, but some get quite cross. I always tell them something my GP once said to me.

'If people need extra time, I give it to them, and as a result the people who are kept waiting know that when it's their turn to need extra time they will always get it too.'

A very sensible outlook on the situation, I thought.

9

In the Community
1991

It had been my dream to work as a community midwife ever since I had attended my first home birth during my training. Meeting women in their own homes gives so much insight into what kind of people they are and their hopes and fears for motherhood. So when Veronica, the community midwives' manager, telephoned me one day to ask if I would like to join the team, I jumped at the chance.

It transpired that Dora, one of the midwives, had decided to start working part-time because she was finding it too difficult to juggle full-time work with the after-school activities of her four children. She agreed to a job share if I could be her partner. I had helped out in the community when midwives had been on sick leave, so Dora knew me and felt we had the same philosophy of putting the women first. I was lucky because I didn't have to have an interview and the position was not advertised; I just started the following month.

It was wonderful. For the first time in my career, I felt truly in tune with the people I was working with. Dora and I were attached to a practice of five GPs who were friendly and supportive, at the same time respecting midwives' specialist knowledge and trusting our judgement. It was very different to working in the hospital, where the women rarely stayed long and it was difficult to get to know them. Now I got to know most of the pregnant women at the practice quite well and enjoyed seeing them through the whole childbirth experience. Of course it wasn't possible to deliver all the babies, but it was nice to look after the women and their families when they came home from hospital.

Dora was a very experienced midwife with tremendous skills and I learned a great deal from her. Unfortunately, even though she always did her best for the women, she did not always see eye to eye with her colleagues. We were similar in that respect, although she was sometimes quite rude and abrupt, whereas I was always careful to be pleasant and charming. I suppose we were both a little bit rebellious in not wanting to bow to the system.

We had avidly followed the developments in maternity practice through our careers. Interestingly, the medicalisation of childbirth was in full swing when I started in the 1970s and that was getting worse in the 1980s, but towards the end of the decade there was a movement back to natural childbirth, led by groups of people who were campaigning against the excessive use of medicine and technology: the National Childbirth Trust, Beverley Beech, chairwoman of AIMS, the Association for Improvements in the Maternity Services for women, and of course Sheila Kitzinger.

Whenever there was a conference advertised in one of the midwifery magazines, midwives from all over the country would descend on London to hear about the latest research in our field. I remember coming back from a conference with my colleagues completely inspired by the movement for more mobility in childbirth, the idea that women should not be made to lie on a bed when giving birth. The boss didn't like it when we encouraged the women to get out of bed, but it just made so much more sense to us. There was another drive to allow the placenta to come out naturally, which takes about an hour, instead of injecting the woman immediately after the birth to speed the process up. This was something else I strongly backed, as I was in favour of as little medical intervention as possible, before, during and after the birth.

I was very excited to hear about the work of Michel Odent, who started the trend for water births over here. It all began in his clinic in Pithiviers, near Paris, where he was encouraging women to give birth under water, because it took a lot of the pain away. Then he came and lectured over here and started a whole new movement. For a while, he collaborated with Yehudi Gordon, an obstetrician working in one of the London hospitals. Their aim was to give childbirth back to women, but some women didn't want it; they wanted to have their epidurals and caesareans, probably because the more conventional doctors felt terrified by the natural childbirth movement's innovations and were discouraging women from trying them.

Even today, if somebody has had a caesarean and they want to have a home birth for their second child, the doctors tend to say, 'You can't do that! It's very dangerous, because the uterus might just split open.' Actually, the likelihood of that happening is less than 0.01 per cent, so why aren't they saying, 'But of course, that doesn't happen to most women'? They never do. They dish out the bad statistics, but they don't turn it around and give you the good ones. I don't think that's fair.

Sometimes new ideas were passed by word of mouth, for instance on study days, when you met other midwives brimming with details about new ways of doing things. Or you would meet someone who had been working in Africa, and she would come and give a talk locally. I picked up information in so many different places! There was always something new coming out and I was always in there, exploring it.

It was great working with Dora, because we both believed in letting women take the lead more in childbirth. We felt it was up to them to decide what they wanted to do. Sometimes they did want to do quite odd things, though. I'll never forget the woman who wanted to sing to her baby as it was born. She was a professional singer and she picked 'Edelweiss' as the song that would greet her baby's entrance into the world. Dora and I were told we mustn't say anything or make a noise, because she wanted the baby to hear her voice first.

So Dora and I sat there in silence as she launched into 'Edelweiss'. It went on and on and on! I couldn't look at Dora, because I knew that if I caught her eye I would start to giggle. When we finally left the house, we burst into fits of laughter. We weren't laughing at the woman, because we really liked her and respected her choices, but it was such a bizarre situation! I still can't listen to 'Edelweiss' now without having a chuckle.

Dora and I had a great partnership and really enjoyed

our work. But inevitably we shared some sad experiences. One that still haunts both of us involved a lovely couple called Shelley and John, who were expecting their first baby just before Christmas. Shelley, who taught children with special needs, had decided she wanted to have her baby in a water pool at home. Their GP, Ian, did not approve of this decision, although he was a great advocate of home birth. He believed that, ideally, people should be born and die within the love and security of their own family home, but because Shelley was thirty-seven and this was her first pregnancy he felt she should give birth in hospital. However, Shelley was absolutely adamant, so Ian agreed to support her and attend the birth.

Dora and I had little experience of water birth, so we accompanied Shelley and John to a special preparation class one evening. This was run by a group of independent midwives, parents who had experienced water births and the owner of the pool hire company. Dora and I were very excited about the forthcoming birth, as we were always interested in new experiences.

When the big day came at last, just a week before Christmas, Dora and I arrived at the house to find Shelley coping really well with her contractions. John and her friend Gwen were with her, giving moral support. It had been agreed that Virginia, another midwife, should come along too, as she had recently been to a water birth and she would be able to give us advice if necessary.

Ian turned up soon after Virginia, with Hilary, a doctor who was training to be a GP, so there was quite a party atmosphere. Shelley and John were in a small room just off the living room, where they had installed the water pool. Dora was with them and the rest of us sat in the living room, chatting quietly. I remember that there was a huge plate of liquorice allsorts on the dining room table for us all to dip into. It's strange how your brain recalls these little details afterwards, but perhaps that's the way it processes traumatic events.

When the birth was imminent, Virginia and I went into the small room to help Dora. All seemed well, until I checked the baby's heartbeat. One minute it was there and then suddenly I couldn't hear it anymore. A look of panic shot between us. It was too late to get to hospital, so Dora sprang into action.

'Shelley, you've got to push really hard now!' she urged.

Some minutes later, the baby was born, a little girl. Dora and I knew immediately that she was dead. I felt a cold wave of dread and sadness roll over me but I didn't have time to dwell on it. I knew on some instinctive level that we had lost the baby, that she had gone, but still we had to do everything we possibly could.

'Ian, bring some oxygen in here, please,' I called out, pushing the door open.

While Ian and Dora started resuscitation attempts, I dashed out of the room to call the Paediatric Flying Squad, which was still in existence then. I knew it was too late, but I desperately wanted the parents to know that we'd fought for their daughter's life. When the team arrived, the baby was taken into the living room, where valiant but futile efforts were made to revive her. Dora, Virginia and I remained in the room with Shelley and John. We had to deliver the placenta and make Shelley comfortable on the little sofa bed. We were all in shock but trying hard to help the parents begin to grasp what had happened. All the words I could think of felt so hopelessly inadequate. Shelley looked exhausted and confused. The full horror had not even begun to sink in.

'Is the baby going to be all right?' she asked plaintively.

'Babies can survive without oxygen for longer than adults,' Virginia replied, rather foolishly.

Dora and I looked at each other and wondered why she had said that, as we both knew the truth. I have always thought that parents should be told the facts clearly and kindly, to spare them the anguish of false hope. Eventually, the paediatrician entered the room.

'I think we should stop trying now,' she said, very softly.

Shelley and John were of course totally distraught and we left them alone together, cradling their daughter, whom they named Ophelia. One by one, everyone else went home, shocked and saddened.

Dora and I stayed for a while and helped Shelley take a bath. She took Ophelia into the bath with her and gently washed her lifeless body. She and John then went to bed and laid their baby between them. I had attended still-births in hospital and, just like this time, I had seen it happen without warning and for no apparent reason. However, I had never before experienced the death of a baby at home. I expected the baby to be taken to hospital for a postmortem, but Shelley didn't want this to happen.

Finally, Dora and I went home. I felt so awful leaving the family there, with this impossible burden of grief. As usual, Derek stirred when I climbed into bed. 'Was everything all right?' he mumbled sleepily.

I burst into tears. Until that moment I had been unable to cry. 'No, the baby died,' was all I could say.

Derek sat up and comforted me until I finally fell asleep.

Virginia told me she had sat up crying too. She lived alone and had no-one to talk to. Her fiancé had died suddenly in her company many years ago and she had been the one to find her father dead some years later. She was completely unable to visit the bereaved parents again, because it brought back her own, unresolved grief.

Ian told me it had been the worst night of his life. He worried that he had lost his skills in resuscitation, because he had not done it for so long. He feared criticism from his colleagues as a result. To his credit, he never admonished Shelley for her decision to give birth at home, but did his best to comfort and support her and John. Would Shelley have been better off in hospital? None of us thought so. But there was no point in thinking about what might have been; it was just too sad.

Our pain was of course nothing compared to Shelley and John's. Ophelia's funeral was held on Christmas Eve. Everyone who had been there at her birth and death went along to her funeral and it was simply agonising. After such a sad affair, none of us felt like celebrating the following day.

Shelley was an extraordinary woman who made me rethink my views on stillbirth. The morning after her baby's birth, she went for a walk with her dog Toby. She took Ophelia with her in a baby sling, because she was not yet ready to be parted from her forever. While walking in the park behind her house, she met a neighbour.

'What happened last night? Is everything all right? We saw an ambulance outside your house,' the woman said.

'I had the baby, but she died,' Shelley calmly told her.

Unsurprisingly, the neighbour was completely traumatised by the sight of the dead baby nestled against Shelley's chest.

Shelley told me later that she had taken photos of Ophelia in the room that was to be her nursery, surrounded by the Christmas presents she had bought for her baby. I began to be concerned about Shelley's mental state and said as much to Ian.

'Don't worry, Shelley is just making the memories that will have to last her a lifetime,' he reassured me.

It made me think how comforting it could be if parents who had suffered the loss of their baby could take their child home for a short time, so that they too could 'make memories'. Happier times lay ahead and Shelley and John eventually had two more children who, while they could never replace the child they lost, have brought them immeasurable joy.

Although it moved and saddened us, Shelley's experience did not put Dora and me off water births, because baby Ophelia's death had nothing to do with being in water. Her heart simply stopped without any warning, which is something that can happen to anyone, anytime. There was no explanation for it and it was certainly not linked to the water birth. It was just one of those awful mysteries of life and death.

Dora and I delivered another water baby soon after that. The woman was in the bath and she decided she wanted to stay there, because she found it relaxing and it helped to take the pain away. 'I think I want to push,' she said after a while.

'Do you want to get out and go into the bedroom, where we've made a little nest for you?' we asked.

'No, I want to stay here,' she said.

'Fine with us.'

She couldn't get her knees far enough apart because the bath was too narrow, so we put her on her side so that she had one leg up in the air. You have to make sure that the water is completely covering the woman, because you can't have the baby half in and half out. It would inhale water that way. If you're going to have water, it's got to be really high and deep, so Dora developed a technique of sticking Blu-Tack in the overflow.

We had read that women shouldn't get in the water too soon, because that can slow the birth down. But as we gained more experience of water births, we found that the women themselves knew when it was right to get into the water, so we preferred to let them decide. Once in the water, their movements were more restricted, so if they were still at the point where they were wandering around and wanting to go into the kitchen to get a drink, they didn't want to get in the pool. Soon we were overseeing quite a lot of deliveries in people's baths, a good while before water births became fashionable.

Ian stoically continued to attend home births and we met up again at the home of a lady called Annika. She had chosen a home birth because she had not had a good experience in hospital with her first child. Her job was designing house interiors and her bedroom was like a photograph from a *Beautiful Homes* magazine. The first thing I noticed, with a heavy heart, was the cream carpet in the bedroom. Would it be as spotless after the birth?

The labour went very smoothly, although at one point Annika and I found ourselves in a very small toilet laughing hysterically about something rather trivial. Annika was using the Entonox, a device that delivers painkilling gas and oxygen, to help when her contractions came – and I think I was probably breathing it in too in the confined space. And of course it's laughing gas! Even the toilet showed off the designer's inspiration. There was a cup and saucer on top of the cistern. The cup was lying on its side and a trail of potpourri flowed out of it into the saucer. I wished I had such talent for home decoration.

The baby was born early in the morning and Ian duly attended when I summoned him. He always liked to be called to home births, even in the middle of the night. After the clearing up was done, Annika admonished him. 'Look, the only damage done to my bedroom is by your shoe polish on the carpet!'

I don't know if it ever did come off!

In 1992, we were given the shocking news that our beloved maternity unit was to close down. This ushered in a period of real disappointment for me. I had been so happy working with Dora out in the community, being based at the unit. I felt I had found my working home, and despite the tragedy of Shelley's baby's death, I was very fulfilled and really felt we were making a huge difference to women's lives. So the news of the closure was a massive blow. It was part of the Government's plan to centralise services, concentrating all the expertise of the medical staff and the technology in one place. The Department of Health had decided to amalgamate our small unit with one the same size in the nearest town. This was terrible news for the small group of staff who worked there. We all had such a good working relationship and felt so much loyalty to the unit. Most of us had given birth to our own children there and some had even been born there themselves! Some of the midwives had childcare arrangements that would be severely disrupted if they had to travel another ten miles or so to work and back. Sadly, many of them were forced to hand in their notice.

The town's residents were also unhappy that the maternity unit was to close, especially as other services were being shut down as well. These included the children's ward, the gynaecology ward and the accident and emergency department. However, no amount of campaigning from pressure groups made any difference. The Government had its way in the end, as it usually does.

If it was difficult for the staff at our unit, it couldn't have been easy for the staff at the new location either. They must have felt they were being invaded. For a time there was a bit of an 'us and them' situation, but eventually the two groups of staff merged and worked together well, making new friendships. The upgraded maternity unit now delivered around three thousand babies a year, so the wards were busier and there was more pressure on the staff.

The NHS had been undergoing continuing change and there were many more managers than before. This created a more structured and less personal environment to work in and the midwives felt that their welfare and that of their patients was no longer paramount. Everything revolved around money. Staff salaries, extra training costs, the cost of patients staying in hospital, provision of baby food and requisites all drained the coffers. Soon the hospital trust was in deficit, which meant the midwives were forbidden even to have a cup of tea when they hadn't had time to go for a break. Understandably, this sort of attitude did not encourage loyalty from staff. What's more, it left them feeling quite disgruntled.

There was a theory some years ago that NHS managers used to be hired from a pool of people who had failed to make the grade in the business sector. Now though, they earned good salaries and their jobs were thought to be quite prestigious. However, the midwives and healthcare assistants still did not earn decent salaries. This was resented by the staff, who felt they were the ones on the shop floor doing all the work, while the managers were sitting in their comfortable offices pushing paper around.

It didn't help that nurses and midwives were now being trained in universities, because now that they had degrees and diplomas, they did not expect to start their working life on low salaries, even if they were doing a job they loved. To me, it doesn't make sense for them to be trained at university. I trained in the school attached to the hospital and we were on a salary, so we were paid for being students. Whereas nowadays, they don't get paid for being a student midwife; they manage on a bursary. During their practical training, they're working all day on the wards, with one or two days a week at the university. They're really working hard and going home at night to study and write essays – and they're not being properly paid for what they do. Sometimes they're even left in charge of a ward.

The new generation of student midwives spend much more time at the university than they do getting practical training, whereas we spent much more time out in prac- tice. I don't think they're getting enough practical training and they don't think they are either, because they say that they don't feel prepared when they qualify. In fact, they're terrified. If they're in somebody's house attending a birth, they could write you an essay on psychology, but they couldn't tell you if or when the baby's going to come out.

The upheavals at the upgraded maternity unit caused a lot of dismay and disruption, but for those of us working in the community, the situation was not so bad. One benefit of the new unit was the inclusion of a birthing pool. This was like a huge bath big enough for two or more people, which was fixed and plumbed in to the water supply. It was different from the portable pool that women hired for a home birth, which had to be erected and filled with a hosepipe.

I was very excited about the prospect of water births at the hospital, but some of the midwives were not so sure. In the event, I was lucky enough to deliver the first water baby. Christine was having her third baby and I had accompanied her and her husband Bob to the hospital when she was in strong labour. I suggested she try the new pool and she readily agreed, even though she hadn't even thought about having a water birth before that. She found the water was an amazing pain reliever and she stayed completely relaxed throughout the labour. When the baby gently emerged, we lifted her to the surface and she took her first breath. She didn't cry but gazed about her with a little frown, as if she was wondering where she was. It was a marvellous experience and Christine and Bob were delighted.

When I came out of the room and spoke to my colleagues, they were interested, but a little apprehensive. 'How did you catch the baby? Did you have to put your hands in the water?' asked one of the midwives.

'No, I fished it out with a fishing net,' I told her with a straight face.

'Did you really?' she said, sounding very impressed.

I snorted. 'No, of course not!'

Some of the midwives never did take part in water births. They were worried about the hygiene aspects, above all, I think, because there's blood and faeces in the water. When you're catching a baby normally, you wear gloves, so ideally you shouldn't get any blood on you. The guidelines are to avoid blood, if possible. You're supposed to wear goggles as well, but I could never bear to. Of course, the gloves only come up a certain way, so you're going to get wet during a water birth. But the women are all tested for HIV, so you should be all right, although there is also the risk of hepatitis. Obviously, we cleaned the pool thoroughly after every birth. It was regularly swabbed for bugs and none were ever detected.

I particularly remember one couple who had planned to

have a water birth. The husband, Max, was an author whose books I had recently read and enjoyed very much. Later, he told me: 'I was so thrilled that you'd heard of me that I phoned my mother straight away to tell her I was famous!'

His wife, Caroline, was in the water pool and Max decided to get in with her. Towards the end of labour, we were all concentrating hard on Caroline's contractions and her breathing. The atmosphere was peaceful but heavy with anticipation, excitement and perhaps a little apprehension. Suddenly, an auxiliary nurse called Betty opened the door of the room. 'Can I take your supper order, Caroline?' she asked shrilly from behind a curtain.

Before I could shush her, she started reciting the entire contents of the menu in a loud droning voice. 'SHEPHERD'S PIE, SPAGHETTI BOLOGNESE, EGG SALAD . . .'

It went on and on. Max and I glanced at each other and tried to stifle our giggles. I jumped up and went over to put my head round the curtain.

'Betty, can you come back later please, we're in the middle of something important here,' I whispered.

Fortunately, the magic of the moment had not been lost and baby David was born into a calm environment shortly afterwards. Later, we all laughed about the incongruity of the situation. 'Maybe I should write a screenplay about life in the labour ward!' Max joked.

They brought me a copy of Max's latest book as a present. Inside the cover was an inscription saying, 'Thank you for the best bath Caroline and I have ever had!'

Water birth became quite popular in our area in the

1990s and I was privileged to attend a really special home water birth one day. When I arrived, Hazel was in labour and being supported by her husband Paul and four close girlfriends. The friends withdrew to the kitchen to make a 'birthday cake' for the new baby, while Hazel lowered herself into the large pool that she had hired for the occasion. Toddler Sarah also climbed into the water, carrying four little yellow plastic ducks to play with. As the labour progressed, Hazel relaxed and breathed easily through each contraction. From time to time, one or other of her friends would appear with a drink, a cold compress or some words of encouragement.

Close to the birth, the ducks kept 'swimming' into Hazel's bump, which began to irritate her a little. Reluctantly she asked Sarah to get out of the water. The baby was born quickly and easily and soon Hazel and baby Robert were tucked up on the settee, with Sarah looking on in awe and a proud Paul taking photos. The birthday cake was brought in with some ceremony, now with the name ROBERT in blue icing on the top. Champagne was opened and everyone joined in the celebration of the birth. I felt so privileged to be part of such a heart-warming ritual, which was something that all the friends did for each other. They were truly supporting the mother and her partner with their empathy, encouragement and practical help. It made me reflect on the stark rule applied in most hospitals: 'One birth partner only allowed in the labour room.'

Another memorable birth happened one Christmas Day. I had agreed to be on call with Marion, a kind and practical midwife who came from the north of England. There were always two of us on call at night for women having a home birth. It was reassuring to have another pair of hands, or just someone to mull things over with, if a labour was going on a long time. It had been hard for Marion to find some-one who was prepared to be on call with her on Christmas Day, as the other girls wanted to be able to enjoy a drink in the evening with family and friends. Still, I didn't mind not drinking alcohol, so I volunteered. It was always better to have a clear head on big family occasions anyway, because my lot plus grandparents and uncles and aunts and nieces and nephews spelled absolute chaos around the house.

In the evening, the phone rang just as my family and I had settled down to watch television after an exciting whirl of present-opening and turkey-eating. It was Marion.

'Right, Agnes, are you ready? I need help here,' she said jovially.

I couldn't believe it: I had just flopped exhausted into an armchair after cooking for twelve people. However, I did feel quite excited – a Christmas baby, just like the Nativity!

When I reached the house, I was a little surprised by the scene that greeted me. Melanie, a young woman who was not expecting her first baby for another two weeks, appeared to be in strong labour. Contractions had started earlier, but she'd thought it was a false alarm. She realised it was the real thing when she suddenly felt an urge to push and her husband Nick decided to call for help.

Since she was visiting her in-laws at their house for Christmas Day, nothing had been prepared for the arrival of a baby. Melanie's own parents and elderly grandfather were also at the house, so it was a real family occasion. Marion had decided there was not enough time to get to hospital, so she was getting her equipment ready for the unexpected event. Melanie and Nick were excited, but understandably apprehensive, and their anxiety was compounded by the sight of two mothers-in-law running around flapping and panicking about the unsuitable conditions for a home birth. The men were very sensibly sitting in the living room with glasses of whisky in their hands.

To try and occupy the mothers-in-law and restore calm and order, I gave them some little tasks to do. 'Could you boil some water for us, please, and collect up some towels?' I asked with a smile. 'And why don't you make up a little bed for the baby? Just improvise with whatever you've got.'

This kept them occupied and they carried out their duties with enthusiasm and plenty of discussion, while Marion and I got on with the business in hand. I presume that boiling water is always called for in films in order to sterilise everything, but thankfully all our equipment comes ready-sterilised in little packets. However, there's more than one use for boiling water – and a nice cup of tea is always a good idea!

When the baby was born, everyone relaxed and came upstairs to welcome him. Great Grandad was absolutely delighted. 'Do you know, ladies, that I was born at home, too, eighty-four years ago?' he told us proudly.

What a wonderful Christmas it had turned out to be for the family, and it had certainly made my day too.

10

Home or Hospital?

The decision about where to give birth is usually made when the mother-to-be attends the antenatal clinic at her local GP's surgery. These clinics are held once or twice a week and run by the midwife attached to the practice. Some women do a lot of research when they find out they are pregnant and express a choice about where to give birth at their first visit to the midwife. Other women need time to discuss all their options and only decide in the last few weeks of the pregnancy.

Traditionally, women tend to visit their GP when they know or suspect they may be pregnant. Midwives are constantly trying to persuade them to visit a midwife first, because it is easier for midwives to give all the relevant information, as they have to be up-to-date with their knowledge of childbirth issues and local policies. GPs are essentially generalists and cannot be expected to know everything about each speciality. So midwives try to see women as early as possible after their referral from the GP.

I really enjoyed these first meetings with the women. It usually took about an hour to give out all the necessary information, answer questions and put them at their ease. For many people, visits to medical professionals are quite scary and they can be nervous or very shy. It was challenging to get them to open up and a privilege when they shared details of their personal lives. Not all women are healthy, well and happy, so this is the time to refer them to other medical professionals, or helpers such as social workers.

Sometimes their partners attended and often they showed great interest and concern. How different to my mother's experience in the 1940s, when men were not expected to have anything to do with pregnancy, childbirth or even child rearing! Except at the very beginning, of course – when for a lot of women the deed was done wearing night clothes, under the covers, with the lights out!

Even in the 1970s, when I started my training, men were not welcomed into the delivery room. They were allowed to view the birth as long as they didn't get in the way or faint, but they were sent outside immediately, well before the placenta made an appearance.

I wonder if things have now gone too far the other way. Should we be encouraging men to stay through the whole experience, from start to finish? Some men are wonderful and can give a woman everything she needs, but that's definitely not always the case. It's not an insult to men to say that some of them need looking after themselves; after all, not all women could give the support required either. A good compromise is to enlist the services of a doula, who cares for the woman, her partner and the whole family throughout the childbirth experience. A doula does not interfere with the medical aspects of the birth in any way, but simply cherishes the mother-to-be and gives loving support, especially during the labour.

If the birth takes place at home, a man who is not able

to meet his partner's emotional needs can at least make refreshments, ensure everyone's comfort and carry out practical tasks. It is not so easy to do this in the hospital, where there is only a small room available to the couple, and so it is difficult for a man to leave his partner in order to restore and revive himself, unless a midwife can be with her all the time. So a doula is a brilliant option in hospital, too. (The word comes from the Greek, meaning 'female servant or caregiver'.) I have worked with wonderful doulas who have not only cared for the parents-to-be, but also for the midwife when she needed it!

Most of my experience as a midwife has been gained at home births. However, I would always support a woman's choice about where she wanted to give birth, as long as she had all the information to make that choice. A woman in labour needs to feel comfortable in her surroundings; if her partner would rather be in hospital, then she will not be happy giving birth at home. Also, there are some medical conditions that require women to be in hospital, as it would be dangerous for them or their baby otherwise.

I have worked with some doctors who tell women unequivocally that they are putting themselves and their babies at risk by opting for a home birth. Once, after I'd arranged for a woman to have a home birth, her GP caught up with me in the reception area of the surgery and said, 'Don't you ever offer a patient of mine a home birth again!'

'Why not?' I asked.

'Because I don't want anything to go wrong. It would be the end of my career.'

How could it spell the end of his career if he wasn't even

there? 'That's a bit biased,' I said. 'You can't tell people that.'

It turned out that his wife had opted for a home birth and something had gone wrong. After the baby had arrived, he had mucus in his throat and turned blue. He recovered very quickly after the midwife cleared his airway, but the poor doctor never got over his fright. It had put him off completely. Subsequently, if one of his patients said she was thinking of having a home birth, he did his utmost to dissuade her.

I disagreed with him, but to no avail. In the end, he really lost his temper. I didn't say anything more; I just walked out, unwilling to be shouted at. The next day I went in and said, 'Can I have a word with you in your office?' Once the door was shut, I said, 'Don't you ever speak to me again like that in front of people! I wouldn't let my children speak to me like that!'

He was very apologetic. 'Agnes, I'm really sorry. I didn't have any lunch.'

'I didn't have any lunch either, but I don't talk to anyone like that!' I said.

Once again, I tried to discuss the advantages of home births with him, by presenting a research-based argument, but with no luck. I respected him as a doctor because he had knowledge and experience and cared very much about his patients, but I could never change his mind about home birth.

Stephanie, one of the female doctors in the practice I worked at, was entirely different. She admitted she was nervous about home births, but acknowledged that it was unfair to turn down a patient's request for one without a valid reason. I asked her if she would like to attend a home birth and she said she would, so I asked one of her patients, Nina, if she would be happy for Stephanie to attend.

It was Stephanie's first home birth and probably one of the few entirely natural labours she had seen. I couldn't help smiling when she arrived and sat stiffly on a chair, keeping her coat on. She was obviously feeling anxious, even though I'd assured her that I wouldn't ask her to do anything because I had a second midwife to help me if necessary. If further help is needed at a home birth, it is more likely to be the specialised expertise of an obstetrician or paediatrician than a GP, in which case transfer to hospital would be required. A GP would not be expected to perform outside their area of normal expertise. Midwives probably have more extensive training in emergency childbirth procedures than GPs, anyway.

Stephanie remained sitting bolt upright in the same chair until it was all over and the baby had arrived. I think Nina was more relaxed than she was, even though she was in labour! But at the next home birth that Stephanie attended, she took off her coat and sat on the floor where I was. She appeared much more confident this time. Juliet, the mother-to-be, had carefully prepared her living room for the birth. There was a large mattress on the floor in the centre of the room and it was covered with a waterproof sheet, with cushions around it. However, when the birth was imminent, Juliet ended up crawling into a small corner of the room, which she made into her own private dark little space. Women quite often do this. I suppose it's very much like how animals behave when they give birth. She had a very calm peaceful birth and was delighted with her new son.

I think Stephanie found this primitive behaviour very interesting and quite different from what she had seen in the labour ward of the hospital during her medical training. She told me she didn't remember much about the births of her own two children, because she had been so drugged with pethidine. She couldn't wait to tell me some days later that she had quite surprised herself by actually suggesting a home birth to one of her patients. She guessed rightly that I'd be extremely pleased with her. She also said she felt she had a special rapport with the babies whose births she had attended.

'I am a born-again GP!' she announced triumphantly.

There will always be some women for whom a home birth would not be a safe option. However, I think it is important to discuss their wishes with respect and honesty and give them all the facts, so that they can make an informed choice. For women in the medical profession, it is often particularly difficult to make a decision about where to give birth. Thinking like a woman, they may wish to have a baby at home, but thinking like a doctor they're more likely to opt for a hospital birth.

One such doctor called Jackie asked me to accompany her into hospital to give birth.

'Oh dear, I'm going to be on holiday on your due date,' I said.

'Don't worry, I know I'll be overdue, so I'll wait for you,' she assured me.

I had delivered her second baby, so she knew me well. When I telephoned her to say I had returned from holiday, a week after her baby was due, sure enough she started getting contractions that night! I do believe that women can delay labour in some circumstances. Emotions and hormones are very closely linked. I have known women whose partners are away on business start labour, then stop, and continue when their loved one walks through the door.

When I arrived at Jackie's house, I found her to be in fairly strong labour. Her husband Henry started to load things in the car. Strangely, Jackie seemed to be putting off going in to hospital, until I told her that if she didn't go soon it would be too late. Then it struck me that she was trying to avoid making the decision to have the baby at home, even though this is what she really wanted to do. Part of her was still thinking like a doctor.

I told her I would support her choice whatever she wanted to do, but only she could make the decision. She then relaxed and resolved to stay at home. I immediately called her GP, Vivienne, because I needed a second professional present and I knew she would love to attend. Vivienne had had a home birth herself, so came at lightning speed and was totally supportive. She reassured Jackie that she was not reckless or a traitor to their profession; baby Carys was born soon afterwards and Jackie and Henry were united in their belief that they'd made the right choice.

One night when I was on call, I met Janelle. Unlike Jackie, she was very keen to go to hospital to give birth to her second child. She lived with her parents and her mother had summoned an ambulance when the labour progressed more quickly than they had expected. Not wanting to deliver the baby in the ambulance, the paramedics had called for a midwife to check on the situation before they moved Janelle. When I arrived I advised her that it would be better to stay at home, because the birth appeared to be imminent. She became hysterical, but her mother's reaction was even worse! A rather flamboyant Caribbean lady, all she could do was flap around, waving her arms and shouting.

'Me husband, he has a heart condition, we can't have no baby born in dis house!'

I tried to calm them both down and was rather glad to see my colleague Diane arrive as backup. The paramedics were also hovering around, reluctant to leave in case they needed to take anyone to hospital . . . and that might well have included Janelle's mum in a state of shock, or her husband with a heart attack!

The baby was duly born into this slightly crazy atmosphere and, once the panic was over, everyone calmed down and enjoyed a nice cup of tea. Janelle subsequently planned a home birth for her third and fourth babies, by which time she had moved into her own house. She definitely became a convert, but I'm not sure her mum approved!

Just as Jackie the doctor had managed to talk herself into delaying labour until she was ready, so did Rosa, who was having her second baby at home. Sadly, her father-in-law had died a week before the baby was due and she very much wanted to attend his funeral to support her husband. She went into labour two days after he had died, but her contractions stopped several hours later. The funeral was taking place a further three days later and she and I discussed what to do. It was being held only about twenty miles away from her home, but because it was on the outskirts of London, the journey might be fairly difficult.

Rosa decided to go to the funeral in the hope that labour would not start until she got home. In the ensuing three days, she had two false alarms, but after a few hours of contractions everything settled down again. She managed to attend the funeral and the gathering for tea at her mother-in-law's house afterwards and travelled home sad but relieved that she had managed to be there. She had only been home for long enough to make a cup of tea when labour started again! This time it continued and the couple's baby son was born a few hours later. Although there was still a lot of sadness, he gave the family a reason to smile again.

One lady called Helen, who'd had a caesarean for her first baby, was very keen to have a home birth for her second child. She was convinced that the way her labour had been managed in hospital had led to her having an unnecessary caesarean. I tended to agree with her, but the hospital's policy was that all women who'd had a previous caesarean section should give birth in hospital. Because of this policy, I was forced to make an appointment for her to see a supervisor of midwives to discuss her wishes. This autocratic manager did not have the insight or empathy to understand why Helen's quest for a normal vaginal birth was so important to her. It meant more than the birth of her baby; it was also about her perception of her femininity and her need to prove that her body could do its job properly.

The supervisor gave Helen some written information about the risks of vaginal birth after caesarean. These notes were not suitable for a pregnant woman to read, because they contained statistics about morbidity and mortality – in other words, the risk of injury and death. I do believe in telling women the truth, but there is a better way to put it than in harsh medical terminology, no matter how intelligent a woman is. Helen was so disturbed by this supervisor that she changed hospitals so that she would not have to see her again, and continued with her plan for a home birth.

When Helen's labour started, there were two community midwives on call who did not feel confident to care for her. They didn't feel they had enough experience to manage the labour and were worried there might be complications from the previous caesarean. I offered to take over, because I didn't want Helen's chance of a normal birth to be compromised. There is a very small risk of the scar in the uterus giving way during labour, but as I've said before, the chances of it happening are minimal. Anyway, there are signs and symptoms which pre-empt it and I felt confident that if a problem arose we would be able to get to hospital very quickly. In the event, the labour, although quite long, was gentle, and a big healthy baby boy finally made his appearance. Helen and her husband Tim were thrilled and I know from our discussions afterwards that Helen felt the scars left by her first experience of birth had definitely healed.

A woman could be forgiven for thinking it would be preferable to have a caesarean section than to give birth to a baby the way nature intended. It can be made to sound so quick and easy and safe. But Eileen, whom I got to know when she had her second baby, was sure that it was not. She had a planned caesarean for her first baby, because he was in the breech position and it is thought to be the safest method of delivery for breech babies. She was perfectly happy, but hoped that when she had a second child she would be able to have a normal vaginal delivery. Sadly, this was not to be, even though her second baby was indeed in a favourable head-down position and everything had been straightforward in the pregnancy.

She had been led to believe that she would have a trial of labour, which means a carefully monitored labour with a specified time limit, so that the uterus is not put under too much strain. But when she went into hospital in the early stages of labour, the locum, or temporary registrar, who was on duty told her that she should have a caesarean section again. There was no basis for saying this at all. I was the midwife allocated to Eileen and, trying to act as her advocate, I argued with the doctor. But to no avail. This misguided man simply insisted on performing a caesarean section.

'If you do not agree with what I am advising, then you can go to another hospital if you wish,' he coldly told Eileen and her partner Robin.

He wasn't really giving them a choice and so reluctantly Eileen was taken to the operating theatre, where her baby was delivered. I felt very angry with the doctor, but he soon went off duty and we never saw him again. Still, the couple was delighted to have their beautiful little girl and Eileen appeared to recover very quickly. She told everyone how fit she was and how she was driving the car just ten days after the birth, going out and getting on with her life.

But she was denying there was a problem. She was trying to convince herself that she was over the emotional trauma, when in fact having the caesarean had affected her badly and made her feel that she was not a proper woman, with a body that had not been able to do what it was designed to do. What's more, she had let a doctor – a man whom she had no respect for, who hadn't even come to see if she was all right afterwards – cut her open and take her baby out. She felt violated. I tried to help her, but no amount of talking to her seemed to make any difference. She could not come to terms with what had happened. Unfortunately, Robin, although a loving partner, did not realise the impact the birth had had on her and underestimated her pain. He cared deeply, but felt she should put it behind her and get on with her life.

Eventually Eileen, desperately trying to prove to herself that she was a real woman, still feminine and desirable, in a moment of madness embarked on an affair. Her lover was part of a couple who were their close friends and, as is often the case, they saw a lot of each other at parties. Friendly banter after a few drinks became sexual innuendo, which then developed into an intimate relationship. Eileen loved her husband, but her emotional unhappiness led her to reaffirm her womanhood with another man.

She soon confessed to Robin that she was having an

affair and he was so devastated that they agreed to live apart for a while. Then, after a few weeks, she came to her senses and realised what she was throwing away. She felt guilty and sorry and finished the affair, begging Robin to forgive her, which to his credit he did willingly. They decided to move house to make a new start and thankfully they remain together. But I know deep down from long conversations we have had that Eileen will never forget the trauma of that second caesarean and the effect it had on her life. If only that doctor could know and understand too. Sometimes doctors seem to think that if a mother and baby leave hospital alive, they have done a good job, but of course there's a lot more to providing medical care than that. Nowadays Eileen would probably be diagnosed with post-traumatic stress syndrome and would be given appropriate help.

Conversely, there are plenty of women who have had to beg for a caesarean because, as the trend for caesareans grew within the medical profession, the Government realised with alarm that an increasing amount of money was being spent on performing them nationwide. They then insisted that doctors justify each operation and give a reason in writing for audit purposes. This meant that, instead of agreeing to women's requests for caesareans, they were denying them. It created a real tension between doctors, patients, managers, auditors and lawyers.

Some women have a real phobia about childbirth. One lady I met was so terrified of labour that she said she would have a termination if she couldn't have a caesarean. Another's mother had suffered three stillbirths and so she was desperate to have a caesarean. I explored all the other options available with these women, gave them all the information they needed and left them to make a decision. If they didn't change their minds, I was happy to support them, accompany them to see their consultant and act as their advocate if they wanted me to. I'm pleased to say that they all got their wish and were convinced that they had made the right choice.

Only one lady regretted her decision to have her caesareans. Briony had worked as an anaesthetist on the labour ward and said she was worried something might go wrong at the birth. She had seen many emergency caesareans performed and was understandably anxious. I could empathise with her feelings as I had worried too when I was pregnant. But I had also seen many normal births and could put my worries into perspective, something it appeared she was unable to do.

Giving birth is often terrifying, whatever age you are, because nobody can really tell you what it's like. I think everybody's frightened; it's normal to be frightened. It would be strange not to be. But it's very unusual to die in childbirth; what I think women are most scared of is being in pain and not being able to control it. Losing their dignity and losing control is what worries most people, even if they know what to expect, and even if it's not a first baby. Nobody wants to be in pain, especially knowing they can't do anything about it. So I suspected that Briony did not want to be in such a vulnerable state because of her professional position.

I was unable to reassure her and she persuaded an

obstetrician colleague to perform the planned caesareans. When I visited her at home after her second baby's birth she was crying. 'I shouldn't have done it,' she told me tearfully. 'Now I'll never know what a normal birth is like. My mum tried to tell me I was making a mistake.' I felt so sorry for her, because we both knew that after two caesareans she would be very unlikely to have a vaginal birth. It has happened rarely, but obstetricians usually don't encourage it because of the risks.

Surely it must be possible to make birth in hospital a less traumatic experience for women? I know it is, because I have seen it done by some wonderful obstetricians and caring midwives. I feel so sorry for women who have an experience they liken to a rape or violent assault. The mother of one woman described her daughter's first birth experience in no uncertain terms when she related what she had been through when she was given an emergency caesarean.

'My daughter was butchered!' she told me angrily.

It is so sad to hear people use words like these about such an important time of a woman's life. Obviously, mothers of daughters in labour are extra sensitive and understandably anxious. It is natural for them to want to do anything to protect their child from hurt. Also, they probably remember their own experiences of childbirth, which may not have been good either.

Sometimes it is badly thought-out hospital policies and protocols that lead to traumatic childbirth. Things are done which are deemed necessary for the wellbeing of the mother and baby, but feel very wrong to the parents, who have often researched aspects of childbirth and are shocked when their plans go awry. But then litigation rears its ugly head and doctors cannot afford to take chances or risks. It should be remembered that in an emergency people's actions can be misconstrued as unkindness or abruptness, when they are simply reacting quite properly to the urgency of the situation.

All these things conspire to cause distress to some couples during what should be the happiest time of their lives. It has been suggested that this has an impact on the parenting of these children and that our whole society may suffer as a result. Whether it's true, I don't know, but I do feel that small, friendly maternity units are much more likely to create a happy environment for giving birth and all it entails. Without a doubt, they can give a more personal service to the patients, while providing a higher level of job satisfaction for the staff.

Huge, impersonal units, where six thousand babies a year are born, may have expert facilities concentrated in one place, but if parents and staff are dissatisfied, then they may not be the best way forward for the NHS maternity service. Obviously, a cost-effective service is needed and provision for high-risk women and babies is essential. But there must be a way of giving appropriate care to low-risk women at the same time as providing emergency backup, without putting everyone together in a high-risk situation.

11

Life After Birth

Many first-time parents-to-be think it is easy to look after a baby. They believe their lives probably won't change that much. Nothing could be further from the truth! When I was nineteen and so young that I didn't know any different, I just got on with it – and by the time I was thirty and on my next lot, I knew what to expect. But most of the couples I have met have found the first few weeks extremely fraught.

Interestingly, the more intelligent they are, the more difficulty they often have. This may be because they have over-researched what lies ahead by reading endless books about childbirth and parenting. They behave as if they are still at work, managing complex projects; they approach parenting as a series of problems for which there are 'correct' solutions.

Sometimes they seem unable to use their maternal and paternal instinct; they insist they haven't got any! And they worry because the baby seems to be awake all night, experiencing a huge sense of relief when they find out this is normal. It doesn't make any difference how many antenatal classes they have attended, they are very rarely prepared for the fact that looking after a baby takes twenty-four hours a day.

Helping women to give birth at home is a small part of being a community midwife. Another interesting and rewarding element is supporting them and their partners in their journey towards becoming parents. It is very satisfying to spend a little time with new mums and dads and help them to cope with their new baby. They have many conflicting emotions, as although they love the baby desperately, they get extremely tired and frustrated when nothing they do seems to settle him or her. It can make them feel quite inadequate.

Older mothers sometimes find it harder than younger mothers, especially if they're used to being in a job where they're fully in control. At work, they know what they're doing, they're in charge and they can plan things. But then a baby comes along and they have no idea what they're doing! It throws them completely and they end up in tears, with no idea if they're doing anything right. It's a nightmare for them. When I came across someone like this, it always made me think back to having Matthew and Edward. I didn't make a big fuss of anything; as a young mum I just got on with it, because I didn't have any expectations.

One of the more commonplace problems that couples experience after the birth is how to make the baby sleep when they want it to. As I've said before, in my opinion babies are like hamsters – nocturnal! And parents can't change that. I advise them to sleep during the day when the baby is asleep. So many times I am greeted at the door of the house by a mother in floods of tears and an exhausted, stressed father. It seems that however much preparation they have, parents have no idea what life with a new baby is like. Many years ago, families tended to live all together or at least in the near vicinity. This meant there were plenty of willing helpers to look after the new family when needed. Now, however, parents frequently live a long way from their adult children and only visit for a short time after the birth. Sometimes this is because the grandparents are still working and sometimes it is because it is simply expected that the new parents can manage on their own.

Asian families I have met seem to have a much better system of family support. Several generations live in the same house and when a new baby arrives there is a never-ending supply of help. The new mother never has to cook or carry out domestic duties; she is treated with reverence and admiration and is looked after until she has physically recovered from the birth.

I believe the media is in part responsible for women thinking they have to get back to normal immediately after the birth. Celebrities are always being applauded for regaining their figures and getting back to work a short time after having a baby. Television advertising shows women appearing slim, glamorous and smiling as they cuddle their perfect, clean and happy babies. The reality of course is completely different, as most new mothers find out. Without the help of those celebrity personal trainers, stylists and nannies, it is impossible to be a glamorous mother, wife and businesswoman! Normal mums can never get those skinny jeans back on, find time to put on make-up or have their hair done. Babies cover themselves with poo and sick just before their mums are due to leave the house. And the upshot of all this is that women feel like failures and get postnatal depression.

I remember visiting the hairdresser after my fourth baby was born. I was looking forward to a treat, because I still felt so fat two weeks after the birth. When I looked at my naked body in the mirror, the image was not flattering, so I thought a sleek new hairstyle would work wonders for my self-esteem.

'When is your baby due, love?' the male hairdresser asked me casually as he combed out my hair.

I was very dismayed by the fact that I obviously looked as enormous as I felt! But I didn't want to embarrass the poor man by telling him the truth.

'Not for another two weeks,' I mumbled awkwardly.

One problem area for new mums is breastfeeding. What should be the most natural thing in the world can cause untold distress to women when it doesn't go right. It can take several days to achieve the goal of a contented mother and baby, but I love to see the look of joy and pride on the mother's face when she at last succeeds with breastfeeding.

Sometimes the community midwives take a student nurse out visiting with them to give them experience of postnatal care. I enjoyed having a student with me because I liked teaching them and it was nice to have company in the car. In hospital, people expect to have students around them and of course are entitled to object if they wish. They may not want a student nurse to be involved in their care; some women may not want a male student to be present. My eldest son, Matthew, is a nurse and by an amazing quirk of fate he trained at University College

Hospital where I started my own training, pregnant with him. When he was training he didn't enjoy his maternity placement at all. He showed enthusiasm and interest but was often excluded from experiences because he was male. I think it can be difficult for male students and that is why I always tried to involve them as much as possible – with the parents' consent, of course.

I don't think people ever expect to be visited at home by students, either male or female, but I have never known anyone to object. I always used to tell the student that if they behaved like a medical professional, the women would accept them as such.

One day I had a male student nurse from Zimbabwe accompanying me on my visits. 'Why do people have so much trouble breastfeeding in this country?' he asked thoughtfully.

'I think it's because most of us don't see mothers openly breastfeeding in public like you probably do in your country,' I replied. 'Goodness knows why, but a lot of people are offended by it.'

It's quite ironic that many women feel perfectly comfortable revealing their breasts in fashionable low-cut tops. Even exposing them completely is acceptable in the media . . . unless it's for their real purpose of feeding babies!

Another male student nurse was allocated to me one day and as usual I asked all the mothers we visited if they minded him being present. I was about to check a mother's stitches and asked if she would like him to leave the room. To her credit, she was quite happy for him to stay. She was sympathetic to his need to learn about what I was doing.

In the car afterwards, I explained to him how stitches in the woman's perineum dissolve. He looked a little bit confused. 'Can I just ask you what a perineum is, please?' he enquired quite seriously.

'It's the area we were just looking at, between the vagina and the anus,' I said. 'You should familiarise yourself with female anatomy during this placement . . . and especially before you acquire a girlfriend!' I teased.

In my experience some men know as much about the female body as some women know about their cars. That is to say, they know roughly the basics of how they work, but there are bits hidden away about which they haven't a clue!

Sometimes new parents have a huge list of questions to ask the midwife. Usually the answers are just common sense, but parents need to be reassured they are doing the right thing for their baby. I believe the media have a lot to answer for, because they constantly give out the message that consumers need to spend huge amounts of money and buy lots of unnecessary products in order to prove they are good parents. One day I visited a GP who had given birth to her first baby two days previously. Her list of questions was two full pages long! And this was one of them: 'Should I use cotton wool balls or buy a long roll of cotton wool for cleaning the baby?'

I couldn't believe that anyone could ask such a ridiculous question, let alone a GP! However, after answering many more such questions very patiently over the course of the next few days, I at last discharged the family. 'I'm going to be a changed GP from now on,' she told me. 'I realise I've been telling women a lot of rubbish about their babies for years,' were her parting words to me. She had realised that new mums would be better simplifying things, especially when it came to cluttering up their homes with unnecessary products.

I was no different to other mums when I had my children. I found it difficult to concentrate and forgot things straight away after being told them. Consequently, I always treat new mums the same, no matter what their job has been. The language I use with some mothers may differ, but the issues I cover are the same.

I always remember the midwife who came to visit me after my third child was born. Tom had developed an unsightly rash that morning, although he didn't appear to be unwell. I was so pleased when Mrs Jefferies arrived, because I couldn't think straight and didn't know what to do. She immediately contacted the GP, who prescribed antibiotics for the baby. I was terribly upset and immediately burst into tears! Mrs Jefferies was not at all fazed by this display, but calmly reassured me that everything was fine and treated me like an anxious mother rather than a colleague, for which I was grateful. Tom had caught an infection during the few hours that we were in hospital, but happily after treatment he was better.

Years later, Fay, the nurse at my dental practice, told me that she had been exhausted and tearful after her first baby was born. Mrs Jefferies was her midwife too, and when she visited she immediately understood the problem. 'Take it easy, love,' she said, 'I'll cook you a nice lunch and look after the baby while you have a sleep.'

Fay was so grateful for this small kindness that she fondly remembered the incident over twenty years later. Another lady I met told me that after her beloved child died, she was very depressed, and Mrs Jefferies had persuaded an acquaintance to give her a little job to get her out of the house. She was definitely a midwife in a million, ever practical and truly dedicated.

Visiting people in their own homes certainly has the potential to create funny situations. Once I was given an address that turned out to be in a labyrinthine block of flats. I eventually found the right number and rang the doorbell; a small child of about three years old answered the door. I told her I was the midwife and asked if I could speak to Mummy. The little girl disappeared and then came back and said I could go with her. I assumed she had been to tell her mummy I was here and that the woman had invited me in. However, we ended up in the little girl's bedroom and she started to show me her toys.

I asked her where Mummy was and she told me she was in the bedroom down the hall. Deciding to investigate, I knocked on another bedroom door. I thought I heard a voice shout out and although I couldn't quite make out the words, I pushed open the door. Mortification! There in the bed were a couple enjoying passionate sex! They stopped, sat up and looked at me open-mouthed.

'I'm so sorry, but your little girl let me in,' I said, covering my eyes with my free hand. 'I'm a midwife, but I'm obviously in the wrong flat.' I don't know which of us was more embarrassed, but I beat a hasty retreat!

Another time I thought I had the right address, again in

a large block of flats. A gentleman opened the door looking rather the worse for wear. He had a can of lager in his
hand and was swaying slightly. 'Are Lily and the baby
here?' I asked pleasantly, not wishing to rile him in case he
was angry at being disturbed.

'I don't know anyone of that name,' he slurred.

'I'm a midwife and I'm looking for a lady who had a
baby yesterday, but perhaps she lives in a neighbouring
flat,' I explained.

He roared with laughter and slapped his rather large
paunch. 'I've got a baby in here and its name is Stella – Stella
Artois!' he bellowed, chortling wildly at his own joke.

I had to laugh too, before leaving to find the real baby.
There was a lot of laughter at the correct address, too, but
this time it wasn't fuelled by alcohol.

But for one couple I visited, there was little thrill and
excitement about bringing their new baby home.
Immediately after the birth, the midwife had told Imogen
and Fergus that she thought their baby may have Down's
syndrome. The midwife herself had a sister with the
condition and she was probably more alert to it than some
other midwives might be. She asked a paediatrician to see
the couple and as he was also concerned about the appearance of the baby, the process to confirm the diagnosis was
put in motion. Blood tests were taken and the samples
were sent to a special hospital laboratory. The couple were
sent home to await the result, which would take a few
days. When I visited the family, they were trying to be
happy about baby Zoe, but at the same time were desperately sad to think of what might be her fate.

'It won't make any difference to us if she has got Down's syndrome; we'll love her anyway,' they told me courageously.

Other family members who were with them that day were quite distraught and there had obviously been a lot of tears shed. I carried out my usual checks on mother and baby and then gave Zoe a cuddle.

'She is really very cute, Imogen,' I said. She truly was a pretty little baby.

If it was difficult for me to know how to handle the situation, how much more difficult was it for the parents? After a few days the results arrived and it transpired that Zoe did not have the condition, so all the worry had been unnecessary. The couple did not feel bitter, just very glad. The only thing that they were sad about was that they had missed out on the chance to celebrate just after Zoe had been born. There was no time to feel amazed, elated or excited, because they were immediately told of the midwife's fears. This, they felt, had spoiled the magical experience of birth for them and they could never recapture it.

Sometimes when new parents express their disappointment about the sex of their new baby, I recall the babies with disabilities I have met. It makes me want to tell these parents that they should be grateful for their perfect child! I can't help thinking of all those women and their partners who can't have a baby at all and who would give anything to become parents. Fortunately, many parents are happy simply when a child is born healthy. I was thrilled when one of my colleagues asked me to deliver her fifth child. She had four girls and when her baby, another girl, was born, she and her husband welcomed her with so much love that there was no doubt in my mind that they didn't care at all about her gender.

For a long time, it was common practice in the area where I worked for ultrasonographers to tell couples the sex of their baby if they could see the genital area clearly. Now this no longer happens, because there is a concern that a woman will ask for a termination if she finds she is expecting a baby of the sex she – or her husband – doesn't want. Unfortunately, this has led to doctors in private practice selling their services to women by offering private scans that will tell them the baby's sex. I find this difficult to comprehend, as I think finding out at the birth is much more exciting. I do acknowledge that I am probably a bit old-fashioned!

This practice of sexing babies is not always problem-free, though. When I met Olivia, she had two boys and desperately wanted a girl. Then, during her third pregnancy, she was told by the ultrasonographer that the baby was another boy, because he had seen a scrotal sac during the scan. Olivia was bitterly disappointed and spent many months trying to come to terms with the fact that she was having another boy.

But when the baby was born, 'he' was in fact a 'she'. What the ultrasonographer had seen was not a scrotum, but the baby's bladder, which appeared as a little pouch outside the abdomen. This fairly rare condition required an immediate operation to put the bladder back into the abdominal cavity, followed by further operations in the future. Of course, Olivia was delighted by her little daughter, who was a lovely surprise. She is determined to give her all the love and care she needs.

12

The Age of Independence
1992

Dora and I had been working as community midwives for about a year when we decided to start an independent practice. This meant giving private antenatal, labour and postnatal care to women, mostly in their own homes. We felt the need to do this because we were frustrated at the way the system worked in the NHS. Although we got to know the women in our care really well, we were not allowed to deliver their babies unless we happened to be on duty when they went into labour. We felt we should be allowed to work more flexibly. But unfortunately our managers at the time did not encourage innovative thought or radical ideas.

So we decided to strike out on our own. We contacted the Independent Midwives Association and arranged to go to a workshop they were holding. It was aimed at midwives like us who were keen to start up their own practice, but needed some practical information and some confidence boosting. What a wonderful organisation we had stumbled upon! We met the most marvellous midwives, who thought exactly the way we did about the medicalisation of childbirth and were trying to do something about it. They were a very forward-thinking group of people, who arranged conferences on maternity issues and managed to get themselves on to various committees, so that they were always at the forefront of any political changes on the childbirth agenda. Most of the members were studying for further qualifications and often wrote articles for publication or even whole books. I felt really inspired by these midwives who willingly gave us so much information and help to get started.

We decided we must advertise our new business and so we asked the local newspaper to include an editorial about us. Unfortunately, this did not produce any clients, only an obscene phone call each! However, we were not going to be deterred.

There was such a lot to think about before we started: What sort of clients would we accept? Where could we buy the equipment we needed? Were we covered by our professional organisation, the Royal College of Midwives, for insurance if we worked privately?

And the most difficult for us . . . How much to charge? Neither of us was comfortable putting a price on the care and support we wanted to give to women, but we had to cover our expenses and pay our accountant, so we couldn't afford to work for nothing.

There were also the practical aspects to consider. If we were still working as job-share partners in the NHS, would we be able to back each other up or would we have to attend births on our own?

Despite all the questions, we took on our first client. Betty was a charming girl whose first baby had been in the breech position and she had therefore undergone a planned caesarean section. She and her husband Duncan were very keen to have their second baby at home, but their consultant had forbidden it. Betty's community midwife had also said she could not agree to a home birth and her superior had supported this view. Betty was absolutely desperate when she contacted us, having heard about us from her local National Childbirth Trust group, an organisation set up specifically to provide information and support for parents-to-be. We had been in touch with them to let them know about our new practice.

We discussed all the issues with Betty and Duncan. The reason the consultant had been against a home birth was his fear of Betty's scar splitting and endangering her and her baby's life. We talked about the research into this issue and how we would monitor the labour. We knew how it was important to be truthful, so that the couple could be in possession of all the facts before making an informed decision. They chose to go ahead with the home birth.

Betty and Duncan were both teachers and did not have extra money to spare for private care. 'Sorry about the deckchairs in the living room. We've forfeited the new suite in order to pay you!' they revealed on our first visit.

This made us feel so embarrassed that we almost gave them free care. However, after a lot of discussion in the car on the way home, we decided that we were providing a service and we had to charge for it. After all, no-one would expect a plumber to work for nothing! We decided we had to toughen up.

It was then that our problems really began. Naively, we thought that if we were open and honest with everyone about what we were doing, they would be helpful to us. How wrong we were.

There is a system in midwifery called supervision. All midwives must have a supervisor who, in theory, is a guide, an advisor and a friend. This also applies to independent midwives, as well as midwives working in private hospitals. It is a system for the protection of mothers and their families, so that they are only cared for by good quality, safe professionals.

A supervisor has the authority to suspend a midwife from practice if she has proof that she is practising dangerously. Managers in hospital maternity departments often become supervisors as well, although these roles are very different. This system of supervision is sometimes abused by these managers, who see it as a way of persecuting independent midwives, because they feel threatened by them. They don't like people working outside the system; they have their protocol and their policies and they like to stick to them. They like all their midwives to stick to them as well, always doing what they're told. Of course, independent midwives don't have to work to those policies. They have to be safe and follow rules, but they have a lot more flexibility.

Midwives must notify their intention to practise to their supervisor in their usual work area every year. If they practise in a different area, the local supervisor must also be notified. This means if a midwife is visiting a friend miles from home and assists a woman having a baby in, for example a shopping centre, the local supervisor must be properly notified of the emergency.

Dora and I were diligent about conforming to this

requirement. Consequently, the local supervisor wrote to us to say we were putting Betty and her child at risk. She also asked the consultant to write a threatening letter to us. She then turned up on Betty's doorstep without making an appointment first. Thankfully Betty refused to let her in!

There was a happy ending when Betty and Duncan's baby son Liam was born in a water birth pool at home, after a short, gentle labour. There were no complications and the couple was delighted. We felt vindicated, but our card was marked with that particular supervisor. Oh dear! It was not to be the last we would hear from her.

A huge boost to our new venture came in the form of a local GP called Isabel. She was planning to have a home birth for her third child and particularly wanted Dora to be with her, because she had delivered her second child. It is quite difficult to be a doctor and a patient at the same time. Of course midwives are the specialists in normal childbirth, but people expect doctors to have expert knowledge as well. It is often assumed that consultant obstetricians, as a courtesy, will see pregnant doctors for every routine check-up. However, many doctors prefer to see midwives, for fear of being unnecessarily medicalised. Isabel understandably felt quite vulnerable, because she had chosen a home birth against the advice of her male colleagues. She needed Dora's reassurance and support.

What normally happened was that whoever was on call would be summoned to any home birth taking place. There aren't many perks when you work for the NHS, but Isabel felt that, as a GP, she was entitled to choose a midwife she knew well. She hadn't reckoned on the auto-cratic management style of our manager, though, who refused to allow Dora permission to attend the birth. So Isabel opted to employ us as independent midwives.

Isabel's husband was a charming man called Tony. He was an accountant and had very little medical knowledge, but he was wholeheartedly in favour of a home birth. The labour started in the early evening and progressed very rapidly. Dora and I had to race to the house quickly and had no time to get our equipment sorted out before the baby suddenly started to appear. Isabel's mother had arrived to look after the other children, so Tony asked if there was anything he could do.

'You can get me some gloves,' Dora said while we were struggling to cover the area of carpet where Isabel was kneeling.

Tony disappeared for a few seconds then tore back into the room brandishing a huge pair of yellow Marigolds – at least they were the rubber gloves, not the flowers! Dora threw them at his head with a snort and pulled a pair of sterile medical gloves from her bag. Poor Tony, he was only following instructions!

Baby William was born a minute later and after Mum and Dad said hello to him, we all laughed our heads off at Tony's blunder. He has never been allowed to forget it, particularly when he and Isabel are socialising with medical friends.

Dora and I met some charming families. One lovely couple, Diana and Martin, booked with us for the births of both their first and second babies. Unfortunately they later separated. This made me sad, not only because I had been through the same thing, but also because I remembered the love they shared during the births of their children. Five years later they were briefly reconciled and during this time Diana became pregnant again. Unhappily, they parted during the pregnancy. Diana was a very strong capable woman with a rewarding career. She decided to have the baby without her husband's support and she promptly booked with us again.

Preparations were made for the birth and Diana's friend and colleague Susie was to be her birth partner. Susie was single with no children of her own and was understandably a little apprehensive about her role as a birth supporter. However, she was a good friend, kind and caring, and Dora and I immediately felt at ease in her company. Being with a woman in labour can often be demanding, stressful and emotionally draining. It is important to give her support, praise and confidence in herself, as well as attending to her physical needs, and sometimes a friend can do that especially well.

Diana was happy for her two children to be present at the birth if they wished. Although they were only six and eight years old, they were delightful and wise beyond their years. They seemed to have an intuitive ability to support their mother.

When the 'birthday' arrived, the house was quite busy. Diana's sister-in-law Ruth was looking after the children in the playroom. The au pair, Anna, and her boyfriend were drinking coffee in the kitchen. Susie and Dora and I were in the bedroom with Diana. From time to time we all changed places. Susie and I would go to the kitchen and Ruth and the children would pop into the bedroom.

The labour progressed slowly and I felt sorry that Diana was going through such an intense experience without Martin. However, when the birth was imminent, we all came together to give Diana the extra support and love she needed. Just at the right moment, Ruth and the children, Susie, Dora and I all gathered in the bedroom and sat silently encouraging Diana to give birth to her baby. As she gently caught the little boy in her arms, there was a look of amazement on the children's faces and the rest of us grinned with delight. There was an almost tangible feeling in the room of the immense power of women being with women. It certainly was a day I shall treasure forever.

Diana continued to bring up the children on her own and Martin sees his new son as much as the other children. Theirs is an amicable and civilised relationship and, to their credit, the children are thriving.

Not all our independent cases were so rewarding. I found one particular woman called Emma very difficult. We never became friends with Emma, as we did with most of our clients. She had one child who had been born by caesarean section and she had never really come to terms with that experience. This time she wanted a home birth, so Dora and I made plans to meet all her requirements.

Unfortunately, she had a long and tiring labour and our relationship became quite strained, as she wouldn't let us help her. She remained very private and withdrew into herself, rejecting our support. Eventually, the baby started to show signs of tiredness as well and I told her that I thought it would be best if we went to hospital. I knew from experience that the baby had become stuck and to delay would put them both at risk.

Emma was adamant that she did not want to go to hospital and said that she felt she needed a bit more time. A short time later, I again said I was concerned, but again she refused to go. The baby's heartbeat was normal, but I knew that could change if it became distressed from the prolonged labour. Also, the scar from the previous caesarean meant that Emma's uterus could rupture if put under too much strain. Although a rare complication, it was nevertheless something that we had to consider.

Emma's husband was a lawyer, so I was careful to ensure that our record keeping was exemplary. The thought of litigation is always in the minds of all health professionals these days. Eventually, as I had feared, the baby's heartbeat began to change, indicating that the situation was becoming more serious.

'I'm not prepared to wait any longer. I'm calling an ambulance,' I told Emma and her husband.

I didn't care what they thought of me then or what the consequences might be. My only concern was to reach hospital and get help. It was decided that Dora should stay with the couple's son who was asleep in bed at the time.

When we arrived at the hospital Emma insisted on walking into the labour ward, rather than sitting in a wheelchair. As I had spoken to the staff while we were on the way, they were expecting us and everything was set up for an emergency caesarean. They were all charming to Emma and her husband; they didn't mention the fact that she had refused to come in earlier. The baby was born with the help of the ventouse. Mother and baby were both fine and to my surprise about an hour later Emma ordered a taxi and they went home!

Unfortunately, I wasn't so lucky and I got a telling-off from doctors and midwives for not coming to the hospital sooner. Independent midwives are not generally well supported by their colleagues and any opportunity to castigate them is usually taken up enthusiastically. On top of this, Emma made it quite clear she was unhappy with my care and the home visits after the birth became quite strained. On reflection, I think she was disappointed with the labour and felt her body had let her down, but she was putting the blame onto me. I was quite happy to let her do so and I looked after her and the baby as well as I could. However, I was glad when we finally discharged her.

I still believe Dora and I did our best and at no time could anyone have found fault with our care. Thankfully, the supervisor of midwives must have thought so too, as we didn't hear from her about the case.

But it wasn't long before the supervisor whom we'd dealt with during our first independent booking tried to cause trouble for us again. We had to notify the supervisor every time we booked a lady in her area, which meant she always knew which women we were looking after. One day, Dora took a lady to hospital after a lovely home birth, because she knew some of the placenta had been retained in the woman's uterus. This is a serious complication that occurs occasionally and can cause the mother to bleed heavily. The treatment is to remove the remaining piece of placenta in the operating theatre under an anaesthetic. So Dora quite rightly took the woman to hospital by ambulance.

The supervisor was of course informed of the patient's admission and scrutinised the woman's medical notes. Record keeping is a very important part of medical care and midwives are always reminded to keep contemporaneous notes and to write very comprehensively during labour care. It is possible for parents to sue for negligence until their child is twenty-one years old; in fact, in the UK winning damages is the only way for parents to receive financial support to bring up a disabled child. Sometimes a child is born with problems caused by an event during the pregnancy that may not have been anyone's fault. Surely a better system would be to award 'no fault' compensation to parents who need money. That way, lawyers would not receive such enormous fees and the NHS might be better off.

So it is understandable that supervisors are always reading case notes and educating midwives about the importance of good documentation. They obviously want to prevent their hospital trusts being involved in litigation. But I don't think this was the motivation behind our hostile supervisor's criticism of Dora's notes when she took her patient to hospital. She laid into Dora for not keeping up-to-date records and said that she should have written notes in the ambulance stating what the condition of the woman was. What the supervisor didn't know was that Dora was holding the baby and the ambulance technician was making general observations on his patient.

The supervisor reported Dora to her superiors, obviously hoping that she would be suspended. But Dora was not suspended when the situation was explained; instead the supervisor was reprimanded for harassment after Dora complained about *her*. And so we were vindicated – and I am pleased to say that particular supervisor has now been demoted after complaints from several other midwives.

My own altercation with a supervisor came when I agreed to care for Theresa and Chris, friends of mine who were expecting their first baby. The supervisor was none other than the antenatal clinic sister from my training hospital, the one with whom I had never seen eye to eye after she told me off for being too familiar with the women in the clinic. After I notified her of the booking, she telephoned the couple and told them they shouldn't employ an independent midwife. Chris found her quite abrupt and rude and he admonished her for harassing them.

When I took my equipment for her to inspect, I told her that I knew what she'd done and that the couple were happy to continue with my care. She realised there was nothing more she could do, but I knew she would be watching me. All went well with the birth and I never saw the supervisor again, but many years later I heard that she had been disciplined for bullying.

A huge problem for independent midwives now is the question of medical negligence insurance. Midwives practising within the NHS are usually covered by the hospital trust for which they work; additionally they can belong to a professional body such as the Royal College of Midwives. If involved in litigation, they would get advice and support, as well as help with their legal fees.

When Dora and I were working together, we had insurance cover from the Royal College of Midwives, so we felt fairly secure. Unfortunately, after a high-profile litigation case involving an independent midwife and the death of a baby she'd delivered, the organisation decided to withdraw this facility from anyone working outside the NHS. We used to have to say to people, 'We must warn you that we haven't got any insurance.'

These days it is impossible to find an insurance company who will provide the sort of cover needed. It's a huge deterrent to anyone wishing to work in independent practice, as it means that a midwife could end up bankrupt and losing her home to pay damages, even if she was blameless. On the other hand, you generally become so close and friendly to the people you take on as clients that I think it's unlikely they'd sue, especially if you haven't done anything wrong.

Nothing much went wrong for us; we were very lucky and generally got on well with the women who employed us. You'd think it would be very well-off women who employed independent midwives, but it's not. Well-off women go to posh, private hospitals to give birth. The women who seek out independent midwives tend to have had a bad experience before and had dozens of different midwives, none of whom they got on with. They want continuity, more than anything, someone who will come to their house and see them regularly before and after the birth.

After working as an independent midwife with Dora for three years, I decided that my career should take another direction. I had always been attracted by the idea of becoming a midwife teacher, and in order to achieve this I needed to embark on a long period of study, because midwifery training was now university-led. I loved having students to teach and was always keen to pass on everything I'd learned during my career, but I felt very strongly that I wanted to have the same academic credibility as the students I was teaching. Obviously, I had plenty of practical experience, but I needed to be able to teach them in a more scholarly way. My contemporaries and I had only been awarded humble certificates at the end of our training, so first of all I had to study for a degree.

I was finding it difficult to look after my four children, spend time with my husband, work for the NHS, attend college and write essays as well as building up an independent practice. Something definitely had to go! Working independently had been a great experience and I had grown professionally, but it had its drawbacks too. I felt constantly ground down with the lack of support from colleagues, supervisors and doctors. It was stressful being on call all the time and trying to keep up a social life with friends. Planning holidays with my family was especially difficult. It was with this in mind that I made my decision to give up.

Dora was naturally disappointed, but bravely decided to carry on and eventually gave up her NHS job to concentrate solely on her independent work. She managed to enlist the help of other independent colleagues when she needed backup and has always remained extremely busy, proving how great a need there is for this kind of service. I continued working for the NHS because I was able to do fixed part-time hours, which meant that planning the rest of my life was easier. At last I could go out with friends on a Saturday night without worrying about being called away to a birth!

13

After Independence
1995

Back working only for the NHS, it was often frustrating having to follow all the policies and protocols of the Trust, especially after being able to work in a more flexible way as an independent midwife. Obviously, there have to be rules for the safety of mums and babies. But sometimes people are so used to doing things one way that they are unable to see that there might be a better way.

And so life and birth went on. During the 1990s, the climate governing midwifery was constantly changing. Litigation was rife, as it was in society generally. Midwives were leaving the profession because of all the stress, and this in turn made the situation worse for the midwives left behind. Childbirth was still too medicalised, despite the protests of women's organisations and campaigns by the National Childbirth Trust.

The risk of litigation meant that more caesarean sections were being performed. In fact, many women were choosing this method of delivery in the belief that it was a safer and easier option. Many women in high-powered jobs couldn't bear the idea of relinquishing control during labour and birth, so they asked their consultants for a caesarean and could then make plans knowing exactly when the birth was going to take place. Women were also opting for epidural anaesthesia, which allowed them to have a pain-free labour. This in turn led to a higher incidence of instrumental deliveries and caesarean sections. Natural childbirth seemed to be dying out and there was no longer any job satisfaction for many midwives. Luckily, we still had women who chose a home birth, so it wasn't so bad for the community midwives.

It was frustrating and depressing to teach antenatal classes and to try to educate and encourage women to give birth naturally, only to hear shocking stories about their subsequent birth experiences. It is difficult to pinpoint exactly what goes wrong sometimes. Time limits are imposed on women and labours are speeded up. A woman can become frightened, particularly if her midwife has to care for several women at once and she is left alone. If a woman becomes stressed her body produces a physiological reaction that is thought may distress her baby. This can result in an emergency which leads to a traumatic birth. Women never forget what happens during birth; I can certainly testify to that. They want to feel empowered by the experience, not traumatised or violated.

The medicalisation of childbirth definitely has a lot to do with the increased use of technology. When I started out as a midwife, there were heart monitors to track a baby's progress, but they weren't used on everybody. Now everybody gets a heart monitor. Fear of litigation is the driving force behind this; there's so much litigation in obstetrics, more than in any other specialty. But we used to find that sometimes the monitors didn't always work properly, or someone misinterpreted the trace. I've seen that happen quite a lot and they've taken the woman to theatre for a caesarean 'just in case'. The woman has to accept this decision, because the doctors warn her that the baby's heartbeat has become irregular. If there's damage to a baby, they are always criticised if they haven't done a caesarean and asked to justify their actions. So now they do a caesarean at the drop of a hat, just because they don't want to be accused of negligence. Yet, as with any operation, there are risks involved. Infection is becoming much more common now after a caesarean than it used to be, so it's not necessarily the best choice.

Amid all the changes and unwanted developments within the maternity service, something that cheered me enormously was meeting my new student, Penny. Aged thirty-three and the mother of four boys, Penny had wanted to be a midwife for a long time, but in the meantime had worked at several different jobs, including running her own business making wedding cakes. It's certainly not easy to look after a husband and children, run a home, work full-time and study, but Penny was very committed and I knew right from the start that she would be an excellent midwife. She and I shared the same zany sense of humour, so we made a very good team, and the patients loved her.

One day Penny and I were at a home birth together. The baby's father, Phil, was a nice man but a drug user and he spent most of the labour asleep in the room next door. Unknown to Penny and me, my Entonox cylinder was leaking and mum-to-be Linda went through three cylinders before we suspected there might be a leak. We then became rather giggly. It may have been the effect of the gas or just the power of suggestion! The baby was born without incident and Dad even managed to stumble in and lie on the bed next to his wife for the event. It was difficult to say who was under the most influence . . . mother, father or midwives!

Unfortunately, shortly after Penny qualified she was struck down with multiple sclerosis. This meant her career options were limited to teaching antenatal classes, as she was no longer able to work on the wards. However, what a teacher she became! The women and their partners were always assured of a good time at Penny's sessions. There was often uncontrollable laughter, especially when she pretended she was in labour and grunted and groaned with great dramatic effect. A stunned silence generally descended over the room and at the end there would be rapturous applause. Not only did Penny help encourage lasting friendships between the couples, she also gave them the knowledge and confidence they needed to give birth to their babies and become loving parents.

Penny and I became firm friends and have supported each other through all the trials and tribulations of bringing up children. We often joked about running anti-pregnancy classes to discourage people from having children that were as difficult as ours!

I finally got my degree, after a lot of hard but worthwhile work. I really enjoyed the studying, and when it was finished I decided to embark on a teaching course straight away, while I was still motivated to learn. On a whim, Penny decided to do the course as well. She took her antenatal class teaching very seriously and constantly strove to improve. Naturally, I was delighted to have her company. I had deliberately chosen to study on a course that wasn't targeted at midwives per se. I thought that if I ever wanted to leave the profession, I could always get a teaching job at a further education college, perhaps lecturing to nursery nurses about baby care.

The first year of the course was spent studying part-time at a local college, along with people from many other walks of life. They were all in various teaching jobs, but had no formal qualifications. It was interesting to listen to them talking about their teaching experiences, particularly as some of them were quite strong characters. One of them taught furniture-making at the local college and another taught languages. Some were quite academic and others more practical. Penny and I were the only medical people in the group.

I thoroughly enjoyed the training, even though I felt that we were not taught about the really important things, like how to manage a class or what to do with troublemakers! I did learn a lot from the other students though, especially when we did a session called 'micro teaching'. This is an exercise where each person has a twenty-minute slot in which to teach the rest of the group something completely different from their normal subject. Their performance has to be videotaped and then their peers criticise them constructively. Penny taught the group how to decorate chocolate eggs to make them into different characters. She appeared to do this quite effortlessly, although she claimed beforehand that she was nervous.

When it came to my turn, I was more than nervous – I was terrified! I was completely unable to sleep the night before because I felt so panicky. I always find it more difficult to stand up in front of colleagues, particularly other teachers, even though they are usually quite kind, rather than being outspokenly critical, as you might expect. I think it's because I strive to be perfect in order not to let myself down. And no-one's perfect!

I decided that my session would be about how to make pancakes for Shrove Tuesday, which fell the following week. My grandmother used to make pancakes for us using her special Scottish recipe and they were always delicious. I made some for the group to taste at the end, which was my way of trying to win them over. I was allowed to take the video home for the night for critical purposes, but I found it so embarrassing that I couldn't bear to let my family see it. I didn't look or sound the way I had thought I would at all. I wondered if actors felt the same way when they watched their own films?

As well as writing various assignments, we did some practical teaching in our own establishment, observed by one of our peers and by our lecturer or one of her colleagues. I taught at antenatal classes and also held individual teaching sessions with student midwives. I found the sessions with the lecturer observing most helpful. She gave very constructive feedback, which enabled me to see myself from the students' point of view. I wrote lesson plans for the first time, thinking through every minute of my sessions in order to prepare properly. I definitely learned to be a more effective teacher as a result.

The second year's training took place in the local university and was more academic and rigorous. Many of the students in my year were members of the police force. Some of them had fairly senior positions and they could be domineering and pushy. Whether this was because of their training, because of the nature of the work they do or because the job attracts a certain sort of person, I don't know. But I had to learn to stand up for myself pretty quickly.

One day I turned up wearing what I thought was a most stylish outfit, with matching red top and red shoes. As I took my place next to Stanley from Scotland Yard, he looked me up and down. 'What kind of message are you giving out today, Agnes?' he said with a sly grin.

'What do you mean?' I asked. I had no idea what he was getting at.

'Surely you know that prostitutes wear red shoes!' he replied impertinently.

Well, I didn't know, but needless to say I never wore them to class again!

After the course was finished, I was offered a few hours' work a week within the local university's Department of Nursing and Midwifery. I was to look after the student nurses during their maternity care placement. These mostly young men and women spent four weeks in the maternity department as part of their general nurse training programme. They had to experience antenatal care, labour, birth and postnatal care, both in hospital and in the community. This was quite a lot to cover in just four weeks. They also had to attend lectures and complete a portfolio of their experiences.

This section of the nurse training programme has since been scrapped and now they have one day with a midwife if they are lucky. It seems a shame, because whatever specialised area a nurse works in there is much that is relevant to general nursing in maternity care. If nothing else, everyone has been born and parented, if not given birth themselves.

My role was to ensure that they made the most of the opportunities available and had a good experience. I had to devise their duty rota and allocate them to midwives who would be their mentors while they were in practice. I used to visit them on the wards to catch up with what they had done and hear about the births they had seen. I really enjoyed my role and made every effort to make these four weeks valuable for their future career.

Some of the midwives viewed the students as a bit of a nuisance, because they were usually quite inexperienced and unable to contribute much to the smooth running of the ward. I tried to emphasise that they would be the qualified nurses and midwives of the future and that warranted the best training they could get. It is easy to forget what it's like to be a student when you have been qualified for a number of years. I think everybody deserves respect, no matter what job they do, and I remembered well my student days when I was considered the lowest of the low!

Later I started teaching at the nurses' study days at the

university. As this was my first attempt at formal teaching, I spent hours and hours in preparation. I had taught small antenatal classes during my teacher training, but now I was teaching about forty student nurses of different ages and nationalities, a much greater challenge indeed.

I took my role very seriously and prepared thoroughly for every minute of the session. I made sure I changed the teaching methods frequently in order to keep the students' attention, because I was well aware of how easy it is to get bored and distracted during a monotonous lecture. I invented games that would enable the students to learn while having fun and I made sure there was plenty of opportunity for them to have group discussions.

Some of these sessions were hilarious, especially the family planning lesson. I brought contraceptive samples with me and there was a lot of embarrassed giggling to begin with. 'Nurses have to be able to discuss intimate problems with patients,' I told the class. 'It's no good falling about laughing when you come across bizarre or shocking things. What would the patients think of you?'

Mostly the students were well behaved and I found it easy to keep their interest if I told them plenty of anecdotes about my time on the wards and community, although obviously I never mentioned any names or gave away any identifying factors. I think that it's always easier to remember how to act in an emergency if somebody gives you an example of something that's happened to them.

There were often nurses willing to share their own experiences of childbirth too, sometimes funny, sometimes sad, and when their stories were sad they always received support from their peers. As many of the students came from the African continent, there were some interesting tales told about childbirth within different cultures. I felt sure this would be useful knowledge when they were qualified and dealing with people of different ethnic origins.

Occasionally I had to reprimand someone, but it was usually in a good-natured way. One student of about nineteen brought a pot of chocolate spread into class. She spent the lesson brazenly dipping her finger into it and licking and sucking with relish! I can't imagine ever doing anything like that during my time in educational establishments. But maybe I'm just old-fashioned! Another student of around the same age came into class, laid her head down on folded arms and closed her eyes. When I scolded her she lifted her head for a second. 'I'm very tired,' she groaned, before promptly going back to sleep!

And what did I do then? I'm afraid I just left her – after all, missing my session would be her loss.

I was responsible for marking the students' portfolios after the course had finished and this was sometimes very amusing. When asked to name a sexually transmitted disease, one bright spark had put down VDU! In computer speak (as I'm sure most people are aware), this is short for visual display unit and I think the lad in question had confused it with VD or venereal disease!

Something I found out during conversations with the student nurses was that they were no longer taught how to give basic care to patients. Cleanliness, pain relief, reassurance and making sure call bells and drinks were within reach were essentials that I was taught as a new student nurse. I was told that these most obvious elements of good care were of little importance now. More time seemed to be devoted instead to computer literacy and essay writing on subjects such as cultural diversity. I believe this is why we hear so much from people about how badly their relatives have been treated in hospitals and care homes. It certainly makes me feel worried, as it may not be too many years before I'm on the receiving end!

Eventually I began teaching student midwives. This meant a lot more academic work on my part, because I had to find and read research before preparing teaching sessions. It was very different from teaching student nurses basic maternity care, but I really enjoyed the job and I loved getting to know all the students. Some were quite young women and others were considerably older, with children of their own. I was still practising as a community midwife at this time but I found it difficult to carry out both roles as conscientiously as I would have liked. Then something happened which made me change the path of my career again.

Among my caseload of patients at the surgery to which I was attached was a young woman called Laura, who was having her first baby. She attended an appointment with me at thirty weeks of pregnancy and her blood pressure was raised. As she had no other symptoms and the reading was normal when I checked it again, I asked her to return the following week. The next time I saw her I had a student midwife with me, who asked if she could run the clinic. I think that because part of my focus was on my student and her training, I didn't really form an intuitive bond with Laura as I usually would, and sadly this caused me to make an error of judgement.

I am not in any way blaming the student – the mistake was all mine – but if I hadn't been trying to do two things at once, I feel I would have been more in touch with my midwife's instinct. This time, Laura's blood pressure was raised again, although there was no protein in her urine sample to suggest pre-eclampsia. However, she did mention other symptoms that I did not at the time believe were relevant, although in the light of what happened they probably were.

I arranged to see Laura at home next to check her again. But the following day, she went into labour and suffered a bleed from the placenta. The baby was only thirty-one weeks and although Laura had an emergency caesarean, sadly the baby did not survive. When the hospital midwife phoned to tell me, I was devastated. I felt it was all my fault and that I should have sent her into hospital earlier. It wasn't clear what had caused the bleed or the premature labour, but it was likely to have been the raised blood pressure.

Despite feeling a cold dread in my stomach, I knew I had to go and see Laura and her husband Simon. I drove to the hospital straight away and found their room. 'I am so very sorry,' I whispered.

Laura went through what had happened, but Simon would not even look at me. I couldn't blame him; I felt, as he did, that I was responsible for the loss of their son. I told them that I was going on holiday the next day but would see them when I returned. Needless to say, I had a pretty terrible holiday. The scenario played over and over in my mind and it was impossible not to think about it.

When I returned home I went to visit them at their house. I thought it would be better to just turn up, but unfortunately I arrived just as they were going out, so we only spoke for a few minutes on the driveway. Again Simon wouldn't look at me, but said they were going to see the consultant to establish whether the care they'd had was to blame for their loss. It is common practice to have an appointment with the consultant a few weeks after losing a baby to discuss what went wrong and what will happen in future pregnancies.

'I believe I made an error of judgement and I am deeply sorry,' I told them sincerely.

Laura said she was not bitter but still wanted to know if the baby might have survived had she gone to hospital sooner. I had seen my manager and, after discussing everything with her, she said she would not be taking any action. I then went to talk to the consultant, who was very kind. He said that if I had sent Laura into hospital, he would not have done anything, as her blood pressure had not been that high. None of my colleagues blamed me but I still blamed myself. I just couldn't come to terms with it. I truly believed I had let Laura down and I could not forgive myself.

My student tried to reassure me. 'You didn't let her down; her own body let her down,' she told me kindly.

I thought this was a very comforting way of looking at

what had happened and I was thankful for her support. But it took several years before I reached a kind of acceptance of the situation. Laura and Simon must have really struggled as well, although I would never wish to compare my suffering with theirs. Eventually they had two more children and both pregnancies went without incident, although I was told by a colleague that Laura's blood pressure was high on both occasions. I deliberately chose to keep out of their way, but I did meet them unexpectedly during the next pregnancy. Simon didn't speak to me but Laura did, for which I was grateful.

I know of other midwives who have experienced incidents like this and each of them has been affected differently. One lied and covered up her mistake, something I would never do. Another left the profession after three of her patients had stillbirths. A friend whose wrong advice led to the death of a baby said she felt some babies were not destined to live, but I'm not sure I believe that or even that she believed it. Still, most midwives who experience situations like these manage to put them behind them and carry on. They just thank their lucky stars if the midwives' governing body, the Nursing and Midwifery Council, is not involved and the patients choose not to initiate litigation.

It was different for me though. What had happened haunted me, no matter how often people assured me that it hadn't been my fault, or reminded me of the risks endemic to working within the medical profession. This was probably the real reason behind my decision to leave my community post and focus exclusively on teaching. As no-one else had wanted to punish me for my mistake, I wanted to punish myself. And at least I would be able to teach other midwives, even if I could no longer practise the job I loved so much.

14

Special Babies and Special Parents

For some people making babies is easy. I never had to try hard myself: the first came along unexpectedly and the other three arrived when planned. But I have never felt complacent and have always been grateful for my luck. I've had friends whose quest for a child dominated their lives and, although I could not know what it was like to suffer like they did, in consoling them I felt I gained a little understanding.

One friend, Sarah, elated to be pregnant after years of trying, sadly miscarried and never achieved her longing to be a mother. As she told me miserably, she had spent years preventing pregnancy when she was younger, confident that she could easily choose to have a baby when she wanted to. I will never forget the look on her face when she bravely cradled my newborn daughter. I cried with her then and felt frustrated at my inability to help her.

Another friend, Karen, and her husband, George, had been trying for seven years to have a second child. Doctors had found no reason for the couple's inability to conceive, particularly as they'd had no difficulty in producing their son. Three years after we met, Karen confided in me for the first time, 'we would desperately love to have another baby and give Oliver a sibling.' Other friends had been having second children when their first were two, three and four and I suppose I'd just assumed that Karen and George were content to have just one child.

I've always thought it impolite and intrusive when people ask about a couple's plans for a family. It is a very private and personal thing and no-one else's business, which is why I had never discussed the matter with Karen. When she willingly confided her worries to me one day, I immediately wanted to help her. She was attending the local hospital where the latest reproductive techniques were not yet available and I felt concerned when she told me that her consultant wished to carry out an operation on her uterus that I knew to be unnecessary and possibly detrimental. I urged her to go to a London clinic that specialised in infertility problems, and which I knew from one of my consultant colleagues had a high success rate.

Karen contacted them straight away and shortly after their first visit, she and George embarked on a course of IVF. This was really a last resort, after extensive tests had proved nothing conclusive wrong with either of them. Karen needed hormone injections at varying times of day and night and I was happy to give them to her. She, in turn, gave me a daily bulletin of how things were progressing.

Everyone was overjoyed when Karen became pregnant at the first attempt. She and George were not rich and had borrowed the money to pay for the treatment, but they felt this child was worth every penny.

I was delighted when Karen asked me to be her midwife.

She was going to have the baby in the local hospital where I worked. After a straightforward labour, she gave birth to a daughter, whom they named Inez. Karen and George were thrilled and I was so pleased to be able to share their happiness. Inez has always been a special little girl to everyone, including her big brother Oliver.

She was born soon after my beloved mother died of leukaemia. My mother had a favourite expression when anyone was feeling low: 'When one door closes another door opens.' So as I've watched Inez growing up, it has always struck me that when the door closed for my mother and her life was completed, another door opened for Inez to begin her life.

I had another friend, Avril, who was also unable to have a second child, but in her case there was a diagnosis. Her husband Peter had been rendered infertile after contracting mumps while she was pregnant with their first child Alfie. At first, Avril was happy to accept that Alfie would be her only child, but when he was five, the desire for another baby completely took over her life. After a lot of discussion and counselling, she and Peter decided that she should undergo artificial insemination with donor sperm.

At that time, sperm was donated by anonymous volunteers. Screened for inherited diseases and their health and well-being scrutinised carefully, they were paid a small amount of money for their contribution on the understanding they did not wish to take any part in the ensuing child's life. The UK law has now changed so that children conceived from donor sperm and eggs can find out their parentage. I am not denying that this is important to a child and I understand that he or she may have a strong desire to know their origins; I also believe that there should be a way of ensuring that donor children do not unwittingly begin a relationship with their own siblings. However, it is no surprise that men are not so keen to donate sperm if there's a chance of being contacted by a child later down the line, let alone having to take responsibility financially or otherwise if the child loses its mother.

Avril became pregnant easily and had an uneventful pregnancy, but she couldn't help worrying because she'd had a traumatic time with Alfie, whose birth had ended in a forceps delivery. She had also suffered from postnatal depression and took a long time to bond with her baby. We discussed a home birth, which I felt might be better for her and for the family in the circumstances. She was very keen on the idea.

I always thought carefully about suggesting a home birth, because I would never want to put a woman or her baby at risk in any way - or, for that matter, compromise myself or my colleagues. I had to decide whether a problem in a previous pregnancy was likely to recur and could always refer a woman to an obstetrician if I needed expert advice. After reading Avril's case notes from her previous pregnancy, I decided it was perfectly safe to encourage her to give birth at home. I was also thinking of her husband Peter and his need to accept the baby as his own child. I thought he would be better able to do this if the baby was born in their home with relatives and close friends around to give him support.

I was honoured that Avril and Peter asked me to be at the birth and we were all excited when her contractions started. She had a long and tiring labour, but handled it with strength and resolve. Peter was compassionate and caring and endlessly patient, especially when Avril became demanding in the latter stages of labour. This phase is known as the transition. It signals the end of the first stage of labour, when the cervix is almost fully dilated, and the beginning of the second stage, when the baby is pushed out into the world. Most women find it a difficult time; some become despondent and think the pain will never end. They shout, cry, are sick or say things that are completely out of character! It is a testing time for the midwife too, as she really has to support the woman and make her believe she will get through.

Peter was a tower of strength and his support never wavered. I couldn't help thinking how he must be feeling, knowing that the baby he would be meeting soon was another man's child.

Earlier, I had called Avril's GP Ian, who had offered to attend as the second professional. It was more usual to have a second midwife present, but a GP could always come instead if they wanted to. Ian had cared for the couple during their struggle to achieve the pregnancy and was keen to be part of the happy ending. After he arrived, he sat quietly in an armchair in the corner of the room.

I began to feel a little anxious, because the second stage of labour was taking rather a long time. I had to consider the possibility that I might need to transfer Avril to hospital if there was no progress soon. Calling an ambulance always felt a bit like giving in, but the safety of mother and baby were paramount.

I gave Ian a look to convey my worries silently; I didn't want to voice them out loud just yet. It is so reassuring to have another professional to mull things over with when a labour is long or difficult. Ian looked calmly back at me and smiled encouragingly, making words unnecessary. The message was that we should carry on a little longer, especially as the baby's heart rate had never deviated from its normal rate. Avril dreaded having to go to hospital, but knew I would not jeopardise her baby's well being for that reason. I knew also that Ian would agree to whatever I decided, as he always claimed that midwives were the experts!

Finally, little Ellie arrived, to everyone's relief and delight. It was touching to see how lovingly Peter cradled her in his arms and kissed her; he obviously had no problems accepting her as his own. He had a large, close, extended family who lived close by and they soon turned up to welcome Ellie into the fold. Within no time, there was quite a houseful. It was clear that Ellie would be much loved.

At her christening, Peter thanked family and friends for their good wishes during their quest to have Ellie. They planned to tell her the circumstances of her birth right from the start and Peter said he knew he could count on everyone's support to help them with this task. Over the years, his love for Ellie has always matched the love he has for his son. Avril was so pleased she had given birth at home and thankfully she bonded with her baby straight away this time.

Many women never achieve their dream of becoming pregnant, despite years of trying. Adopting babies these days is less common than it used to be, because single mothers are supported by the state and there is little or no stigma now. Finding a surrogate mother to have your baby is also difficult. I have met a few women who have managed to have a child of their own by this method and it is wonderful to see their joy when cradling a baby in their arms at last. I admire the altruism of the surrogate, as for me it would be the most difficult thing in the world to give a baby away, whether or not the child were genetically mine.

Of course, there isn't always a happy ending when a couple wants a baby. Ailsa and her partner Sandy lost their first child Maisie at the age of six months because of a heart defect that could not be corrected. They had another child called Angus a couple of years later and thankfully he was healthy. When the time was right they decided he should have a playmate and Ailsa became pregnant again.

Unfortunately, she suffered a miscarriage, but they were determined to try again. She had no difficulty in conceiving and the fourth pregnancy was soon underway. Because her first child had been born with a heart defect, she was sent for a specialist ultrasound scan to check all was well this time. Sadly, it was not. The scan detected that the baby had a serious heart problem, which although not the same as Maisie's, was inoperable. What's more, it meant the child would not live after birth.

Ailsa and Sandy were distraught and after a lot of discussion with the obstetrician and paediatrician agreed to a termination of the pregnancy. The baby was already fully developed and they saw it a part of their family, so this was not an easy decision to make. Some people may think it better to continue with the pregnancy and let nature take its course, but it has to be a couple's individual decision as to what is right for them.

After a period of grieving, Ailsa and Sandy agreed to have one more try. Once again, Ailsa became pregnant easily and was duly sent for a detailed scan of the baby's heart. This was carried out in a specialist unit in London. When, to their absolute joy, everything was pronounced fine, the couple felt immensely reassured. At last they could look forward to achieving their dream of completing their family.

With four weeks to go before the baby's due date, Ailsa attended her midwife's clinic for a routine antenatal check up. However, her midwife was dismayed when she detected an unusual heartbeat; she arranged for Ailsa to be admitted to hospital straight away. Ailsa and Sandy awaited the arrival of the consultant with trepidation. After monitoring the baby's heartbeat, performing a scan and conferring with colleagues, he made his decision. He could not be sure what the problem was, but he thought it best to deliver the baby by caesarean section as soon as possible.

This was a shock for Ailsa and Sandy. Everything had

happened so quickly that they had no time to gather their thoughts or prepare themselves for what was to come. The baby, a boy later named Rory, was born gravely ill and transferred immediately to an intensive care unit in London. Sandy accompanied his son, but Ailsa had been given a general anaesthetic and so it was a while before she was awake enough to be given news of her child.

Tragically, Rory died some hours later, before she was able to say goodbye. Sandy returned to the hospital to tell her about their son's last hours and for days they remained inconsolable. Still, they were not bitter that Rory's heart defect had not been detected; it was something they simply accepted. Unaccountably, it was a different condition to Maisie's and their last baby's.

They were so devastated that they resolved never to risk another pregnancy and Ailsa was sterilised some months later. Ailsa was one of six children herself and none of her siblings had lost babies or had children with any problems, so perhaps the combination of hers and Sandy's genes was at fault. Of course, Angus is a great blessing to the couple as he has given them so much joy. But despite having a successful business and plenty of material wealth now, nothing will ever make up for the loss of their four babies. Ailsa, to her immense credit, channelled her grief into raising money for charity and counselling other bereaved parents.

Losing a baby at any stage is devastating and having a still-born baby is a terrible tragedy. A midwife colleague talked to me after she lost a baby. 'I don't know what to say when people ask if I have any children,' she said sadly.

'It might not be something you want to discuss with a mother-to-be, but why should you have to deny your child has existed?' I replied, 'You are still a mother and your baby will always be a part of your family, even if she has died. So I think it is all right to say you have had a child.' How painful it must be to work as a midwife when you have lost a baby yourself. I have so much respect for the people who are able to do so.

Some people have huge obstacles to overcome before they even try to get pregnant. One couple I met in their early twenties had their own special challenges. Carla had been born with cerebral palsy and used a wheelchair. She had only limited use of her limbs, her movements were jerky and her speech was unintelligible except to the people who knew her well. Mentally, she was of normal intelligence. She was married and her husband Ewen had a mild learning disability that prevented him from working.

Carla and Ewen had been living in an old peoples' home, which was most unsuitable for them, but they were pleased to have recently been allocated a council house on an albeit rather rough estate near the centre of town. It wasn't a great location for them because the estate housed known drug dealers, prostitutes and troublemakers and I couldn't imagine them getting much neighbourly support there. But they would rather that than be in the old people's home.

I first met them when they came to the surgery where I was holding a clinic. Ewen had pushed Carla's heavy wheelchair for over a mile uphill, so I said I would visit them at home in future. When I arrived at the house, the local health visitor was there. 'Whose idea was it to have a baby?' she asked them sharply. 'How do you think you will manage to look after it?' I thought this was unnecessary and discriminatory, but Ewen was quite confident in his reply.

'We think we'll get on OK, I look after Carla, don't I?'

It was true that Ewen was Carla's sole carer; he dressed her, fed her and carried her to the toilet. So I understood the health visitor's concerns, although I think they could have been voiced more sensitively. I just hoped that more help could be provided for the couple after the birth.

Carla's body was so twisted that she was booked in to have a caesarean section. I was a little anxious that the operation might endanger her health, but my worry proved unfounded and their little girl Tia was born healthy, despite being a few weeks premature. When my visits to them came to an end, they seemed to be coping well and were thrilled with their daughter. One can only hope that Tia's childhood will be happy and that she will not end up being a carer for her mother.

I have met several deaf mothers and because of my hearing problems I feel a special rapport with them. Iris used sign language with her family, but she could lip read and speak a little. Her preferred method of communicating with hearing people was to write things down. I always used to visit her armed with plenty of sheets of paper for our discussions. It made me realise how much I rely on tone and inflections of voice to express myself. Hopefully, the way I speak can put people at ease and show them I'm friendly and empathetic, but giving the same impression is much more difficult in writing. I tried to smile a lot and use gentle touch on the arm instead.

Iris' partner Clive was also deaf and so were their three children. When they were all together and signing it seemed like a normal household with children…except silent. I admired them all so much for being able to lead a normal family life within a society that is definitely not sympathetic to their hidden disability.

I have also cared for blind and partially sighted women and am always struck by their courage and how they manage to look after their families. I suppose they have to be very organised and know where everything is in the house. But how difficult that must be when you have children. My teenagers' bedrooms always looked as though they had just been burgled, as their possessions were always flung around everywhere!

I met a lovely lady called Tania who was expecting her fourth child. She had lost a leg in an accident, but was always smiling and managed to look after her family as well as run a successful business. I laughed when she told me she had thrown a jug of water over her husband after the birth of her third baby in hospital; a bad reaction to medication had made her act in a mad way. This time the birth was to take place at home and I made sure she had no drugs, although her husband kept out of the line of fire anyway!

I will always remember her sitting up in bed after the

birth, wearing an enormous pair of sunglasses. She looked like an eccentric movie star! I didn't like to point out that, as well as being indoors, it was the middle of winter! 'Don't take away the water,' she said with a chortle. 'I'm not really nuts, I've got a bit of a headache and the glasses help.'

Physical disabilities can be a huge hindrance to child bearing and rearing; it can be fraught with problems for those with mental health issues. One such lady called Frances had been diagnosed with bipolar disorder some years before I met her. This condition used to be known as manic depression, but is now much better understood, although treatment is not always successful. Frances was under the care of a psychiatrist and a mental health nurse, but did not need medication as she was on the less serious end of the bipolar spectrum. An intelligent single woman in her thirties, she had accidentally become pregnant by a man with whom she was no longer in a relationship. She was determined to do her best for her much-wanted baby and her family were very supportive.

Frances told me about her mental health issues from the start. She was very knowledgeable about her illness. I was duty bound to make a report about her to the midwife responsible for child protection, who oversees a wide range of cases and problems that might affect the well-being of a baby. Domestic violence is another common reason for her involvement. Consequently, social services were duly informed about Frances and an appointment was made for her to be seen by a social worker.

It is important that we all work together to achieve the best outcome for a family, so I promised Frances that I would be there to support her. At first the social worker was rather patronising in the way she spoke to Frances. However, when Frances explained about her condition and added that she had a degree in psychology, the woman hastily concluded the interview, satisfied that all was well. I came to like Frances very much, even though she was quite needy during the pregnancy and wanted to talk at length at each of her antenatal appointments. She constantly required reassurance. I found it easier to see her last in my clinic, so that I could devote more time to her.

Eventually the baby was born after a long and difficult labour that was overseen by a sensitive and compassionate midwife. Frances went home the next day and appeared to be coping well. But on the following day, baby Billy became very unwell and Frances called her GP. When she was told that the doctor would not visit until lunchtime, she called an ambulance and she and Billy were taken to the accident and emergency department of the local hospital.

Once the staff found out that Frances was bipolar, their focus changed from Billy to her. The nurse and doctor insisted that this was a feeding problem and that she was just an anxious mother. Frances lost her temper and created a scene, because nobody would believe that Billy was really ill. After several hours, they were finally seen by a paediatrician, who immediately recognised that the baby was definitely poorly. He told her that Billy had a serious infection and that if she had not acted when she did, he could easily have died. They were then transferred to the paediatric ward of another hospital where there were better facilities for sick babies.

All this took its toll on Frances, who was stressed and upset, a state which she tried to avoid in case it brought on her illness. I visited her in hospital after she phoned to tell me about her ordeal. I felt sorry that she had been so alone during her struggle to make people understand that, even though she had a mental health problem, like any other woman she still had a mother's instinct. What the consultant had said absolutely vindicated her; thank goodness she'd had the strength and courage to stick to her guns.

I spoke to some of the nurses that day and was surprised at how little understanding there was of bipolar disorder. I came across the same ignorance in some of my colleagues, a few of whom were actually quite worried in case they were asked to visit Frances. It is hard to be physically different in this world, but perhaps even harder to be mentally different.

In the course of my work, I have come to realise that there are all sorts of families, with all sorts of problems and complications, but as long as there is plenty of love, difficulties can usually be overcome.

15

Those Who Can, Teach
2000

When I trained, midwives used to be taught on the wards by senior midwives, as well as having some periods of study in the school of midwifery attached to their hospital. I certainly felt that I was adequately prepared for the job, but midwife training had changed radically since then.

I have known several women who are not so academic, but are compassionate and caring, practical and sensible. In other words, they would make excellent midwives. But this opportunity is now denied them, as the entry requirements to the course are A levels or an Access course, both of which demand a fairly high level of academic ability. However, whether this was right or wrong, I still looked forward to my new role teaching student midwives, as I really wanted to make a difference to their training. I wanted to teach them new skills and be a good role model as a midwife.

I enjoyed teaching very much, even though I got terrible stage fright. I think it must be comparable to acting, because I prepared, I rehearsed and I watched other people do it – and then I felt a great sense of achievement when it was over! I knew that students could be very critical and rather cruel in their judgement of me. After all, I'd been a student myself once. Even if a teacher was good at their job the students would find something else to laugh at, like their fashion sense!

I was quite sensitive because of my eye abnormality and I was always anxious to prove that the rest of me was normal! My other problem was that my hereditary hearing loss had steadily been getting worse, so interactive teaching sessions were quite difficult for me. I had to try to sit students in a way that meant I was able to walk up to them if I was unable to hear a question. I explained that I wasn't trying to intimidate them by standing so close; it just made it easier for me to hear them.

Whereas the students didn't seem to find this a problem, my colleagues weren't quite so accepting. I suppose I was a bit of an outsider, because the other lecturers in the department had on average twenty years of teaching experience and not much practical experience. But I had the opposite.

I found the university system difficult to understand at first and there seemed to be a lot of internal politics to deal with. There were endless meetings at which I was always one step or more behind everyone else, because I found it difficult to hear everything that was said, especially when voices were raised and people talked over one another. As a result, I wasn't able to contribute much to the meetings and presumably people thought I was a bit dim. Unfortunately, this is always one of the hazards of being deaf. There was also a lot of paperwork to contend with, so the actual time spent with the students was very limited.

The lecturers themselves were an interesting bunch of people. They were obviously highly academic and some of them spoke in something I got to know as 'lecturer-speak'. This consisted of English words but sometimes with an Americanisation – and used in an order that didn't make any sense to me! They would also say things like 'I hear what you're saying' and 'I'm taking that on board and thinking outside of the box' and sometimes they would 'flag things up' or 'run this up the flagpole'!

The head of the department, a lovely lady whom I admired and respected, always spoke in a very unaffected way in her naturally pronounced regional accent. I confided to her one day that sometimes I wasn't sure what the other lecturers were talking about and she unhesitatingly reassured me. 'Don't worry,' she said with a grin. 'They do it deliberately so that people will think they're tremendously clever!'

That not only made me feel better but also made me determined to speak plain English. I told my hospital colleagues that if they ever heard me using 'lecturer-speak', they should knock me out and shut me in a cupboard until I'd got over it! They assured me they would. Still, some of the lecturers were very helpful and supportive to me and I learned a lot about teaching from them. Others, however, were rather patronising about my lack of teaching experience. The most senior lecturer, on learning that I had a hearing problem, asked me, 'Why don't you stay at home and be a housewife?'

It makes me laugh now when I think about it, but it does make you wonder. Hadn't she heard of the Disability

Discrimination Act? Perhaps I should have reported her to a higher level of management; after all, the university always stressed its commitment to giving equal opportunities to staff and students. At the time, though, I just shrugged off her words and got on with the job.

Some of the midwives treated me differently when I became a teacher. They became a bit deferential and acted as if I knew everything, which of course was ridiculous. I told them I might know where to find information, but I certainly wasn't a fountain of knowledge, and I wasn't any different now I was a teacher. I made sure that I mucked in with everyone else when I was on the wards. I really believed we could teach students most effectively if we all worked together.

The midwifery training itself concerned me too. There was a lot of academic work – too much, I felt. Of course, it is important for students to understand the theory behind the practice and know how to access research. But I wondered how ready and able they felt to actually become midwives.

Some recently qualified midwives confided to me that they felt anxious and unprepared for the practicalities of the job.

This could have been because, as students, they didn't spend enough time in clinical practice or maybe the practice they experienced was not the most helpful sort. They told me that they had learned that birth was a natural life event and that a woman's body was designed for childbirth, with hormones finely tuned to ensure the whole physiological process took place naturally. Any interference or attempt to speed things up was likely to cause more problems. However, interference was what they regularly witnessed. The well-meaning obstetricians tried to take control over childbirth and in doing so often inhibited the process.

The students found that they were often caring for a woman who'd had an epidural anaesthetic for pain relief so they never learned to recognise the natural rhythms, behaviour and breathing that take place during birth. Some women really needed an epidural during a long and difficult labour, but many others did not. In some cases, it can be positively detrimental to the birth process and increases the risk of an operative delivery, in other words a caesarean, or at the very least the use of a ventouse or vacuum extractor. The natural way may be more painful at the time, but often it's easier for mother and baby to bounce back after the birth than it is when there is medical intervention.

Student midwives had to deliver forty babies during the course of their training and it was often very difficult for them to do this when so many women required an operative delivery. It would definitely have helped if they had been called to home births, as there were a higher number than the national average taking place in the area. However, many of the community midwives were quite possessive about their women and were reluctant to let a student deliver the baby, whereas I don't think it matters who actually catches the baby; just being with the woman is the important part.

The midwives used to say that the woman herself asked

that her midwife and not the student should deliver the baby. However the woman, especially if she is on all fours and not facing the midwife, often doesn't know or care whose hands are poised. I have met some wonderful midwives who encourage the mother to lift up her own baby so that only her hands touch the baby. I often encouraged it too, but only if the mother suggested it first.

Our practical teaching sessions at the university were always a lot of fun. Sometimes they were on important topics, such as how to manage emergency situations. They took place in the practical skills training department and the technician who supplied the required equipment was an amiable man called John. He was a bit like the props person in a theatre production. As well as dealing with all the latest computer presentation technology, he often had to nip out to the local supermarket for the oranges we used for demonstrating injections. He had to supply fake urine for testing – he assured us it was fake and not his own! And he also supplied copious amounts of realistic-looking blood. The role-play we used for managing a haemorrhage after birth involved bags of this blood. A teacher would lie in bed pretending to be the patient and would puncture the bag at an agreed moment. Then the students would be called in two or three at a time and would be tested on whether they coped calmly and properly with the scenario. Even though I always hated role-play as a student, I had to admit it was a good way to learn practical skills, because it was easier to remember than a straightforward lecture.

* * *

I continued teaching for a couple of years but soon I was longing to get back to clinical work. I missed the mums and babies so much. All the lecturers were supposed to put in several hours of clinical work each week, but this was extremely difficult to do. Lesson preparation, marking, tutorials, meetings and masses of administration always seemed to get in the way. For the first time I felt admiration and sympathy for all the teachers I had met at my children's schools over the years. I certainly never appreciated how much work was going on behind the scenes.

Something else that made me want to return to being a community midwife was that I frequently met former patients who said they missed me. I lived in the same road as the doctors' surgery where I used to be based; the local school was also nearby and I used to see lots of mums with 'my babies' walking to school in the morning. We always waved to each other as I passed in my car. I often met mums in the supermarket and sometimes it took a long time to get round and pick up my groceries because I liked to have a chat with each one. In the end, my husband decided not to come with me anymore, because he would inevitably be left to do the shopping by himself, while I admired all the babies!

So eventually I made the decision to leave the university and go back to clinical practice. I didn't regret the time I'd spent teaching, as it had satisfied a desire I'd always had; I knew I could do it and I loved it, even though it was nerve-racking at times, and I felt I had a real rapport with the students. I would continue to mentor students on a one-to-one basis, so I didn't feel like I was giving up teaching completely.

I also had an extra little teaching job at the time that I thoroughly enjoyed. I ran a couple of sessions a year for a group of men and women from various foreign countries who were training to become interpreters for the hospital trust. They were all proficient at English, but needed to know specific medical terms, diseases and treatments in order to be able to work in a healthcare setting.

I found these people very interesting and they often had quite a lot to say about the NHS. Some claimed to have better systems in their countries, where the standard of living was not as high as that of the UK, but the care was superior, they claimed. We could have discussed these issues in depth, but my role was to familiarise them with everything to do with the maternity care experience. Still, I think we all learned a lot from each other.

Another kind of teaching that I always enjoyed was running antenatal classes for parents-to-be. In the 1970s these comprised a straightforward lecture by a midwife, with questions invited at the end. Then a physiotherapist might teach some complicated breathing patterns for labour. The couples were then shown a video of a rather medicalised birth. A patient wearing a hospital gown and lying on her back in the labour ward bed would be producing a baby quietly and cleanly in a sterile environment, while her masked and gowned husband looked proudly on. The film would then cut to the couple enjoying a nice cup of tea while the baby slept peacefully in the cot beside them.

Over the years, these classes have completely changed and evolved. The main purpose of them now is to provide parents with a weekly meeting place, to enable them to make friends and form their own support network. The sessions are supposed to inform them about the birth process and alleviate any fears they may have; they also encourage the parents to start family life with confidence in their parenting skills.

I have taught many different kinds of parents-to-be over the years. The sessions for teenagers were always a challenge. These young people had a very short attention span and it was important to keep them entertained and occupied. For some of them, lack of money and no partner or family support would mean life with their baby would be a tremendous struggle. It was important to give them self-esteem and encourage them to help each other.

There were also classes for mums-to-be only, for women on their own or those who wanted to go while their partners were at work. I always enjoyed these, as they usually turned into a good old girly gossiping session! Well, as long as everyone gained something from the classes, the format wasn't important. And I liked to encourage the women to share their worries and feelings with each other.

The most difficult classes for me were the couples' sessions. In the area where I taught, there were many middle-class people who often had quite well-paid jobs in the city. They would get home from work in the early evening and have to be at the class by 7pm, maybe not having had time for a meal. They were often a fairly dynamic group of people, accustomed to both giving and receiving slick presentations during the course of their working day. I had to make sure I kept their attention, gave them what they wanted and encouraged them to enjoy themselves.

Interestingly, when they arrived for the first session, the ten couples always came in looking rather apprehensive. They didn't know each other and they sat around in a circle, not speaking to anyone other than their partner. I think this is a peculiarly English trait. Commuters can travel on the same train to work every day with the same people, but if they haven't been introduced they never speak. It was my goal to have these couples chatting like old friends by coffee time halfway through the first class. To achieve this, I used various tried-and-tested methods. I didn't want anyone to feel threatened or embarrassed by having to speak to the group, so I usually asked people to chat in fours to start with.

I remembered going to study days as a newly qualified midwife and having to introduce myself to a group of people. I was so petrified that I could never listen to anyone else, because I was concentrating so hard on what I was going to say – that awful feeling when your mouth goes dry and your heart thumps in your chest! I certainly didn't want to put anyone through that. I judged the success of the classes on whether the group became firm friends a few weeks later. I encouraged the mums to meet for coffee every week after the sessions had finished, until all their babies were born. This was exciting, because one by one they dropped out of class and whoever was missing was presumed to have given birth. Years ago, the mums or dads would phone each member of the group and discuss their birth stories. With the arrival of the internet, now they usually send an email to everyone and often include photos of the new arrival too!

I remember two particular couples for an unusual reason. Hayley and Mick were two sixteen-year-olds who were excited about their expected baby, even though they hadn't planned the pregnancy. They were the youngest people in the room, but they were intelligent and eagerly participated in discussions. They were very much in love and because their parents gave them a lot of help, they were hoping to be able to support themselves and their baby well.

The other couple, Vanessa and Stephan, were in their late thirties and had been trying to conceive for several years. Vanessa was a journalist and Stephan was a consultant child psychiatrist. They were expecting twins, thanks to in vitro fertilisation or IVF, the wonderful discovery which has helped so many women to have babies. Although Stephan worked with children, he admitted that he knew very little about babies.

It so happened that Hayley and Mick had their beautiful baby daughter, Rachel, the week before the series of classes finished. To my delight, they came along to the last class with Rachel; everyone admired her and was anxious to hear the details of her birth. During this discussion Rachel needed her nappy changing, so Mick very dexterously popped her onto a changing mat and expertly got on with the job.

While he was doing this, Stephan questioned him about his technique. 'You look so confident handling Rachel,' he said. 'I hope Vanessa and I can do as well as you!'

This made Mick very proud of himself and Hayley very proud of him. It made me think what an interesting scenario this was and how teenage parents should not be stereotyped, but judged on their own merit.

I used to enjoy organising reunions for the new families, which were usually held about six weeks after the last class. This sometimes took place in one of the couples' houses, if anyone had enough room for ten couples plus babies! If not, then in summer they met in the very pleasant local park and in winter in the children's area of the local pub. I was always invited to attend these gatherings and it amused me to see that the dads were the ones holding the babies all afternoon. When joining in their conversations I would hear lots of talk about nappies and baby behaviour. A sign of the New Man, no doubt! Sometimes the men arranged a night out on their own with their new friends and sometimes the women went out and left their partners babysitting – lads becoming dads. Sometimes they all met up together. I have often bumped into people while shopping who have told me that their group is still meeting up more than ten years later! I felt so proud of the part I had to play in these lifelong friendships.

16

Back out in the Community
2002

When many of our local hospital services were closed down, including our beloved maternity unit, it was a great loss for the community. The maternity areas had recently been refurbished and a brand new, million-pound operating theatre had been built, but then not used. We all wondered why this huge amount of money had been squandered and who was responsible. Although we understood that changes are often good and can improve services, we all felt a great sense of betrayal.

Local pregnant women also had to adjust to travelling far longer distances to have their babies. Of course, anyone living and working in the Highlands of Scotland or remote areas of the West Country would think eight miles was a very short journey, but it was a difficult transition for people in the area used to having their own hospital.

One positive result of the move was that there were more home births. This was very rewarding for the community midwives, who all enjoyed attending them. Sometimes mothers also had their babies at home unexpectedly, as they had left too little time to get to hospital. One charming lady called Verity had previously endured two very long labours and resigned herself to the fact that her third baby would drag on for a similar length of time. She had made arrangements for her children to be cared for while she was in hospital and had prepared little snacks to keep her husband Stuart well nourished during the marathon labour.

I was having a lie-in one Saturday morning, leisurely reading the papers, when Stuart telephoned me. I wasn't actually on duty that weekend, but my number was the first one he had found in his panic. He urged me to come and see his wife because she seemed to suddenly have a lot of pain and said she felt like pushing. I jumped out of bed, threw on some clothes and raced up the road to their house. Fortunately, they only lived a few minutes away. When Stuart opened the door, he looked quite white and he led me up the stairs to the bedroom where Verity was making grunting noises. I reassured her that everything would be all right.

'Can you bring me my equipment out of the boot of my car, please?' I asked Stuart. A beautiful baby girl was born five minutes later to an astonished but elated mother. Dad and children were very excited and I later left them all together, happily awaiting the arrival of the grandparents. I was delighted to have had my Saturday morning lie-in curtailed in this way! The birth also had a bonus outcome for me, as Stuart happened to be a plumber and I was able to call for his assistance when we had a serious leak in our attic one day. Well, he couldn't really refuse, could he?

Every labour is different and I learn something new at every birth I attend. A very unusual thing happened during the birth of one of my colleague's children. Daisy had just finished her training to be a midwife after practising as a nurse for many years. She had then found herself unexpectedly pregnant with a fourth child and had decided to have the baby at home. Her husband was not very supportive of the idea, but as she had given birth to the last two children at home she persisted with her plan. I was flattered when she asked me to care for her and we talked about the sort of birth she hoped for. Right on time she went into labour and I made my way over to her house after she telephoned me.

She progressed fairly quickly to reach nine centimetres dilatation of the cervix, but then nothing more happened. The cervix or neck of the womb has to open to ten centimetres before a woman can push the baby out. I knew the baby was in a posterior position with his back against Daisy's spine and his face looking up instead of down. Babies who lie like this often take longer to make their way through the pelvis and can sometimes get stuck. But I wasn't worried because Daisy had managed to have three fairly straightforward labours before.

Well, we waited and waited and still the contractions didn't abate. I knew they were painful. Daisy's youngest child, Flora, aged ten, was comforting her mother and holding her hand. Guy, Daisy's husband, wandered in and out, looking rather at a loss. I had called for my assistant midwife Marion a while before, thinking that the baby would soon be born, but no such luck. A little later, the baby began to show the first signs of distress and I immediately made the decision to transfer to hospital. Daisy was disappointed but knew she needed help.

The ambulance turned up very quickly and Marion and I climbed in with Daisy while Guy and Flora followed in the car. Unfortunately, we had to travel down a single track road for a couple of miles and the drivers of two cars that we met had to be asked to reverse to the nearest lay-by to allow us through. They weren't very happy about it either, despite the very obvious flashing blue light! How can people be so thoughtless? Eventually we arrived at the hospital after a fast, bumpy ride. Sally, the driver, was magnificent and negotiated roundabouts, crossroads and lunatic drivers with extreme skill. I never want to hear anything detrimental about women drivers again!

When we arrived at the hospital the baby's heartbeat was monitored and he was no longer showing signs of distress, but even the jogging around during the journey hadn't shifted him. He was still stuck and Daisy's cervix was still not fully open. The registrar who was on duty wanted to start an intravenous hormone drip to try to speed the labour up. But I was worried that Daisy's uterus might rupture if he did so, because the contractions were so strong and frequent. After a discussion with the consultant on call, it was decided that a caesarean section should be performed.

By this stage Daisy was begging, 'Please just deliver the baby. I've had enough!'

Hours of painful contractions and the journey to hospital had taken their toll. Unfortunately, there was a locum anaesthetist on call who had a great deal of trouble inserting an epidural catheter for the anaesthetic. He refused to resort to a general anaesthetic or to call a senior doctor for help, but at last, after what seemed an interminable length of time, he succeeded and the operation began.

Freddie, a big, healthy, bouncing baby boy weighing in at ten and a half pounds, finally entered the world! Guy and Flora were waiting anxiously outside the theatre, and when they heard the news their faces showed enormous relief. Marion and I felt emotional too and some time later, over a cup of coffee in the staff room, discussed what had happened. It had been a very unusual scenario and we concluded that Daisy's age – she was forty – along with the laxity of the pelvic floor and Freddie's size and position had probably all played a part in his getting stuck. It again made me realise that a midwife can't ever afford to be complacent, because you never know how things may turn out.

During the next few weeks, I was asked to help out in the community in the neighbouring town, because they were short staffed. I was quite happy to do this and it meant that I would be seeing quite a different sort of population. The people there were not so affluent and there were many more single mothers living in pretty basic accommodation.

The first time I attended a home birth with Marie, the local midwife, she told me off for taking my shoes off when I arrived. 'Better keep them on; you never know what you might tread on in this house!' she guffawed. However, the family, although not very clean, were lovely people and had a lot of respect for midwives.

The next time Marie called me to a birth, I had to go to

a block of flats in the town. It was the middle of the night and Marie had instructed the woman's sixteen-year-old daughter and her boyfriend to wait outside for me, flag me down and show me where to go. When we all entered the block of flats, there were several young people hanging around the hallway, despite the late hour. They were drinking and who knows what else. As we went up the stairs to the flat, there was loud music coming from the living room and youngsters of various ages wandering around. I wasn't sure who lived there and who was just visiting.

The woman in labour, whose name was Tracey, was in the bedroom swearing and shouting. Marie was with her. Tracey's partner, Dan, was sitting on a chair and another daughter of about fourteen was perched on the bed. From their conversation, I gathered that Dan was not the girls' father and this was a new relationship. Tracey was not being very pleasant to Dan. She seemed to be blaming him for all the pain she was in and calling him some rather choice names! This may have been helping her to get through the contractions, as sometimes shouting is quite therapeutic.

'Keep quiet, Tracey, or you'll frighten the neighbours,' joked Marie.

'F*** the neighbours!' spluttered Tracey.

Quick as a flash, Dan retorted, 'Yeah, you've done that already!'

It was hard not to laugh. Presumably there was some sort of scandal involving Tracey and a neighbour, but Marie and I didn't ask. The baby was eventually born and everyone calmed down; the whole family and all the onlookers appeared to be genuinely pleased. We could only hope that the baby would be brought up in a loving atmosphere, whatever the circumstances.

Next, I met a very nice lady called Wendy, who was expecting her second child. She'd had a bad experience during the birth of her first baby in hospital: a doctor had treated her in an uncaring manner and spoken to her quite rudely, prompting her to complain. Her husband, Nigel, had been on his way back from abroad and only got to the hospital after the baby had been born. Wendy felt the doctor would have been different if her husband had been present and Nigel felt guilty that he hadn't been there to protect his beloved wife.

I suggested that this time they might like to have a home birth. I encouraged Wendy to do her own research, talk to friends and ask me any questions she came up with. Some weeks later, she and Nigel decided to go ahead. But when the labour day came and I visited them to assess things, Wendy seemed troubled. She was definitely in labour, but when anyone was in the room with her the contractions stopped. I think subconsciously she was reliving the previous bad birth experience and her body was not allowing labour to continue. I left her alone in her bedroom and chatted to her sister who was staying to support her.

After some hours there was still no progress, so I told Wendy I would go home, as I felt my presence was putting her under pressure. I suggested that perhaps she and Nigel should just relax, have a cuddle or even go for a walk. Sometimes we suggest sexual stimulation, as the hormone activated by arousal is also the one needed for labour.

Although Wendy's cervix had opened up halfway and second babies can suddenly come very quickly, I felt sure this would not happen. This was really a last resort before having to go to hospital for the labour to be speeded up. If labour lasts too long, the baby may become tired and the mother's energy can deplete. However, I was keen to avoid the hospital because of Wendy's previous experience.

A short time later, Nigel phoned to say the contractions had started again and were much stronger. They had done as I suggested and it had worked. I returned to deliver the baby and soon mum and new little son were happily tucked up in bed together. Wendy told me a few days later that she intended to become a midwife herself and I'm thrilled to say she eventually did.

Another interesting experience I had was with a lady called Naomi. The first time we met, I could see she was a very troubled young woman. I had ten patients to see that morning at the surgery for antenatal checks and they were each allotted ten minutes. This was obviously not going to be enough for Naomi, though. She told me she was expecting her second baby and she did not appear to be completely happy about it. I gently probed into whether she had any worries.

'I had an absolutely dreadful time having my first baby and I'm really frightened this time,' she confided.

I coaxed her to tell me what had happened. In the back of my mind I was worrying about the rest of the women waiting outside, but I decided that if I didn't help Naomi now, she might never open up to me again. It was obvious that she was ready to talk about it, probably having psyched herself up for the appointment, and I didn't want to let her down by sending her away without having listened to her story.

She looked at the floor. 'I had a long and painful labour and the midwife was unkind and unsympathetic. I had a forceps delivery and an episiotomy that took six months to heal properly.' She added that she had felt violated and it seemed as if the baby had been dragged out of her, while she was made to lie passively, wracked with pain.

'I couldn't bond with the baby for months and I suffered from postnatal depression, which lasted for ages,' she went on. 'My husband Rick and I had no sex life at all for a year.' This had understandably made things difficult for them, even though they loved each other.

They eventually felt able to plan another child, but when Naomi found she was pregnant all the bad memories came flooding back and she became terrified of giving birth again. I thought it would be a good idea to consider a home birth so that Naomi would not have to go to hospital and be reminded of her previous trauma. We could also make plans for a very different experience this time, which we would work together to achieve. She went home in a happier frame of mind and we arranged to meet again soon to discuss things further. I felt privileged that she had trusted me enough to tell me about her anxieties and I resolved to help her to the best of my ability.

The next time I saw Naomi, she seemed a bit more positive. She had talked to Rick and he liked the idea of a home birth. I was sure he too was traumatised by what had happened to his wife, something he admitted when I got to know him a little better. Naomi and I talked about the reasons things may have gone wrong before and strategies for overcoming problems this time. It seemed that at the start of labour, baby Joe had been in a posterior position, otherwise known as back to back, and this had made the experience long and painful. So we discussed how to get this baby in a better position using simple techniques like keeping the knees below the pelvis and adopting forward leaning positions when relaxing at home in the evenings. A very clever midwife called Jean Sutton, who had a background in farming and engineering, devised these techniques to help women avoid an operative delivery.

We also worked on Naomi's attitude and I encouraged her to be positive and believe in her own body's powers. She loved scuba diving and said how much she would like to have a water pool, so this was arranged. Eventually she seemed to be really looking forward to the birth.

When she went into labour one evening, she telephoned me, sounding excited. 'Hi, Agnes! I'm getting contractions, but they're not too painful and I'm coping at the moment,' she said.

I went to her home to assess her and check the baby's condition and we decided that I should leave her for a while. 'Just call me and I'll come back when you're ready to get into the water pool,' I said.

When I returned to the house after Rick phoned me, Naomi's contractions were quite strong and ten minutes apart. Rick was being very supportive and, although obviously worried himself, he was as kind and loving as he could be. Naomi was ready to get into the pool and I had to call another midwife, as the rule was that there had to be two of us when a woman was in the pool.

Naomi's mother was staying in the house to look after Joe and she was a tower of strength. The water worked very well and Naomi progressed very quickly, to the point where she withdrew into herself and concentrated hard on getting through each contraction. Sometimes I wiped her brow and gave her sips of water and sometimes Rick took over. None of us spoke much, so as not to disturb the unique concentration needed for this mammoth task. Occasionally, I would gently stroke Naomi's arm or hold her hand, whatever seemed appropriate, just to let her know I was truly with her and to try to give her strength and confidence. She became very empowered. She knew she was in charge and was no longer frightened or anxious.

Eventually she whispered, 'I'm ready to push!'

And to the strains of some haunting classical music, we watched in wonderment as the baby slipped gently out into the water. I helped Naomi to lift her up and as she clutched her to her breast, tears of joy silently trick-led down her cheeks. The baby opened her eyes and calmly looked around, then blinked as she gazed at her mother's face. Rick tenderly kissed his wife and they smiled at each other before laughing in delight at what they had achieved. I knew then that Naomi had been healed and that this birth had made up for the trauma she had suffered previously.

In the days that followed, when I visited the family, Naomi told me how much she had enjoyed the experience. Although she had been in pain, she'd felt calm and strong and in control. It is at times like these that I think this is what midwifery is all about and I wish all midwives could take part in a birth like this.

One not so happy birthday took place on the day I returned from a month-long holiday visiting my son, Edward, and his wife in Australia. I always find the first few days back at work to be a bit disorientating; to add to this, I was in the middle of a very busy clinic when I had a phone call from the hospital to say a lady was giving birth unexpectedly at home. Apparently, there were no spare midwives to attend her, so I had to abandon my clinic and rush away. The women were very understanding and either saw a GP or made another appointment. The receptionist told them that I had to go to someone in an emergency and one lady said she felt very reassured to hear it.

'It's good to know that any one of us will get help urgently if we need it,' she said.

When I arrived at the block of flats, an ambulance was already there and two paramedics were with the couple. Gloria and her partner Vincent were known to be drug addicts and Gloria's first child had been taken into care by social workers. There were also domestic violence issues. When problem cases such as this are identified, all the midwives are notified. Gloria was supposed to be going into hospital for the birth, but her labour had been very rapid and the baby had been delivered by the paramedics. The little boy was four weeks early and quite small; I now had to persuade Gloria to go into hospital with him in case he developed problems. Babies who are more than three weeks early can develop breathing or feeding difficulties or be unable to keep warm. This little fellow was going to have drug withdrawal symptoms as well.

Gloria knew that if she went to hospital her son would be taken into care. If she stayed at home it would be more difficult to accomplish this. So at first she argued with me and Vincent became quite aggressive, but eventually I got them to agree and I accompanied her in the ambulance. I felt incredibly sorry for her, because surely nothing can be worse than having your baby taken away, but at the same time the safety and wellbeing of the baby were paramount. I had to put the child first. Of course, the inevitable happened and the baby was sent to foster parents as soon as he was well enough. A very sad case, and all too common, I'm afraid, but the little boy was safe and that's what counts in the end. I sincerely hope that Gloria can be helped to turn her life around. She and her children deserve a lot better than their current situation.

17

New Hopes
2003

In 2002 there was more bad news for our local midwives
and mothers-to-be. The hospital in the next town, which
had served our population since our own local maternity
unit had shut down, was itself to close. There was a sense of
disbelief and despair among the staff; for some midwives
this was the third time their jobs had been relocated. We
were told that services would be transferred to a bigger
general hospital several miles away. The new large obstetric
unit would have to deliver about six thousand babies a year.
I felt resigned but I was still upset. I had been watching this
process of centralisation gain momentum throughout my
career. Despite all the work that had been done to show that
home births can be safe and beneficial for mother and baby,
the constant restructuring of the NHS meant that in practice, maternity departments were getting bigger and bigger
and birth was getting increasingly medicalised.

There was one ray of sunshine. To offset this huge blow,
the staff were told that it might be possible to open a birth
centre within the old hospital. This would be a maternity
unit run by midwives and, although it was on the hospital
site, there would be no obstetricians or paediatricians
available. This meant it would only be for mothers with

straightforward pregnancies and no risk factors. Anyone with a history of problems or certain medical conditions would be excluded. It would, in effect, be like having a home birth and the criteria for booking would be the same.

Birth centres incorporated into obstetrics units of large general hospitals were opening up all over the UK. These centres were run by midwives who had the security of knowing that a fully equipped delivery suite was only a trolley ride away. There are women who would not wish to give birth at home, but are quite happy to have a baby in an isolated or 'stand alone' birth centre – and not only because they're worried that something might go wrong. Some people have neighbours who live close enough to hear through the walls! Some live with their parents and would not have any privacy, or they live in mobile homes with very little space and no shower facilities. Others have animals that roam around the house and would get in the way of a home birth.

I have seen at first-hand how home births can sometimes be a bit of a challenge for these very reasons. I once attended a home birth where a huge dog lay at the feet of its owner, Ursula, while she was in labour. Ursula's bedroom was very small and moving around meant climbing over the dog!

Accompanying me to the birth was Gill, the practice nurse from the local surgery. She knew Ursula as a patient and had asked her if she could attend. 'I never saw a birth during my nurse training, so it would be a great experience for me,' she told her. Ursula generously agreed. The dog was not mentioned.

What no-one knew was that Gill was terrified of dogs. She stood stock-still in a corner of the room throughout the labour in the hopes that the huge animal wouldn't notice her. Meanwhile, I was worried that the dog might want to eat the placenta when it was delivered, having read that this is what animals do in the wild to deter predators. I wasn't scared of the dog like poor Gill, but I didn't think it was very hygienic to have it acting as a birth partner. All was well in the end – no-one got attacked and nothing inappropriate was eaten!

On another occasion I attended a woman called Zara, who had planned for her birth to take place in her perfectly adequately sized bedroom, but actually crawled into the bathroom when the time came. No amount of coaxing would persuade her to come out and she crouched in front of the bath while her husband, Luke, sat inside it. There was no water in it at the time!

My student midwife, Jo, was squashed between the toilet and the bath, poised to catch the baby. My colleague was wedged between the door and the radiator. I had to sit on the toilet, as there was nowhere else left. I did put the lid down first! It was quite a small bathroom and not built to accommodate five people – well, six if you count the baby – some of whom were quite large (well, the mother was nine months pregnant . . .) It was like a bizarre game of sardines!

So there are a variety of reasons why women might choose a birth centre over their home. These small units are very popular with midwives too, as they have free rein to practise the real art and science of midwifery within them. Since there are no doctors, there are no epidurals or caesarean sections. Anyone who develops complications is transferred to the nearest obstetric unit. Occasionally, a woman may ask to transfer if she wants an epidural, but this doesn't happen often. Women who choose a birth centre are usually confident they will manage. They can expect one-to-one care there; with so much support, they usually cope well with the labour.

This is not to say that choosing a fully equipped obstetric unit is a mistake; women should give birth where they sense they will feel happy and positive, even if there are no complications. Some women are very afraid of labour and worry that something will go wrong. This is probably due to the way birth is portrayed in society now. Of course, unexpected complications can always arise, but it is a question of putting the risk in perspective. You don't refuse to travel by car in case you have an accident! Statistics for birth centres are very carefully audited and results have proved to be good.

Many midwives like birth centres because they can really be 'with woman', which is what the word midwife actually means. Some midwives feel they get more job satisfaction from caring for one woman holistically than from running between two or three on a busy delivery suite, where they probably have to talk to doctors, answer phones and do numerous other tasks as well.

Many of the midwives at the threatened maternity unit didn't believe that our birth centre would ever become a reality. They had been lied to by management before; why would they trust them now? Two senior midwife managers were sent to our unit to oversee the transfer and smooth things over with the staff. These women were very dynamic and motivated and promised that they would get a birth centre up and running if it was what we wanted. So all the midwives who were interested got together and formulated a plan. This covered the criteria for booking, as well as all the various policies and protocols. Also to be taken into account was the building work required to convert the hospital labour ward and the training that the staff would need to extend their skills.

In the meantime, I got myself a part-time bank contract at a birth centre that had already been set up about fifteen miles away. I wanted to see how a birth centre was run and use the experience to advise the team planning our own unit. Working as a bank midwife means that you have a flexi-time contract with the employing NHS trust. It's ideal for midwives who have children and cannot work regular hours. It also means they can take the school holidays off if they need to. The disadvantages are that they receive less holiday pay and no salary if they are sick. Also, work is not guaranteed, so for some people a permanent contract and regular income are preferable.

From the Trust's point of view, employing bank staff is better than hiring agency midwives to cover shortages, because they are cheaper. Agencies charge a fee for their services and also pay their staff more money. This means, of course, that it is more lucrative for midwives to work for an agency than to have a bank contract. It's a huge problem for the NHS, which loses staff to agencies all the time. This could be remedied if the trusts paid their own staff more money and offered them better benefits, but for the foreseeable future the current policy is contributing to the crisis in midwifery.

The midwives in the birth centre were a very friendly and committed bunch. They worked autonomously and really supported each other. The women attending the centre were very different to the sort of women I encountered in my own area. Living in the Home Counties, in a town that was a commutable distance to London, meant property prices were sky high. It followed, therefore, that most of the women I met were affluent and middle class. At my new job there was a great ethnic mix and people with varying levels of income. Their cultures and religions were all different and this made the work very interesting.

The midwives treated the women as partners in their own care and everyone was shown the utmost respect. Although there were no doctors on the premises, there was a very supportive consultant attached to the local hospital who was happy to see any woman with suspected or actual problems.

I loved working at the birth centre, but I wasn't entirely happy about how much support was available in a crisis. If I called for help on my own patch, I knew I could expect a colleague to be with me within about five to ten minutes – or perhaps a little longer in the middle of the night. Indeed, an ambulance would usually arrive in even less time. Here, though, I wasn't so sure that the backup was in place.

One weekend, I was the only midwife on duty, along with a maternity assistant called Lisa. These assistants had positions of great responsibility. Their duties were answering the telephone to prospective users of the birth centre and discussing whether they met the criteria for booking. They welcomed and showed around parents-to-be, students and midwives from other areas. They were responsible for ordering stock and carrying out clerical duties, such as entering data onto the computer, and they had to clean and prepare the birth rooms. Most importantly, they assisted the midwife at a birth if there was no second midwife available. For this they received the lowest pay grade that existed for untrained staff. The women undertaking this role were dedicated and highly motivated and obviously not doing it for the money.

I had just been saying to Lisa that it looked like it was going to be a quiet day when we had a phone call from a distressed father-to-be. He and his partner had arrived in the hospital car park; she was in strong labour and couldn't get out of the car. I raced down the corridor, pushing a wheelchair, and made my way out into the car park, where I spotted a young girl puffing and panting. I managed to persuade her to get into the wheelchair and raced her back to the sanctity of the birth centre. Her waters had broken and we left a trail along the carpet as we went. As she climbed on to the birth room bed, I could see the fluid was a greeny colour, indicating that the baby might be in distress. Thankfully, she shouted that she wanted to push and I encouraged her to do so.

Just then, Lisa came into the room with some suction equipment and oxygen. 'Lisa, please call an ambulance and try to get a second midwife to come in,' I asked quietly.

The reason for this was that the baby had opened its bowels inside the womb and passed meconium, an unborn baby's faeces, which is sometimes an indicator that the baby is compromised. Even more worrying, there's a danger the baby may inhale the meconium, which could cause breathing problems. I was concerned that if I had to transfer the baby to the nearest special care baby unit, I would need an ambulance as well as another midwife to take over from me at the birth centre.

The baby was born after a couple of pushes and to my intense relief cried straight away. She was in excellent condition, so the most likely reason for the meconium was the rapid delivery, which could have left her a bit shocked. Anyway, all was well and the ambulance was cancelled. Lisa told me later that she had been unable to contact a second midwife.

We all settled down to have a cup of tea when, unbelievably, the phone rang again and another woman in a similar situation arrived in the car park! I couldn't believe it and neither could anyone else when they saw me running down the corridor with a wheelchair again. This time we got back to the birth centre in time, but I only just managed to get the woman's trousers off before the baby made his entrance, crying lustily. This birth was straightforward, thank goodness, and when all the parents and babies were settled and the paperwork was completed, we finally got to have our cup of tea. From then on, whenever I saw that stain on the carpet, I thought of that day and all its drama. As it happened, it was Mother's Day . . .

*   *   *

Eventually our own birth centre opened, as promised, and it was a popular choice for many women. It was a poignant moment for me, because I recalled how, in the 1980s, there had been a similar unit in one of the towns nearby. It was known as a GP unit, as some of the local doctors enjoyed participating in normal childbirth, and it was situated in the grounds of a cottage hospital that had no emergency facilities and no permanent specialists. As anyone who has worked in the NHS for years will tell you, trends dictate changes in how you care for people, but it happens quite often that you end up working in a revamped equivalent of something that used to function perfectly well years before.

One day there was a tragic incident at the GP unit involving a woman who was in labour with her second child. She'd had a delivery with her first baby, using Keilland's forceps, which were designed to turn a baby's head from a posterior to an anterior position if it was stuck high up inside the vagina. They were an unwieldy piece of kit and could easily cause damage to the mother's delicate tissues and to the baby's head, so much depended on the skill of the operator. Their use has largely died out now in this country. If a baby is in a posterior position and the baby's head is too high for a vaginal delivery, a caesarean will usually be performed.

In hindsight, Eve should never have been booked to give birth at the low-risk GP unit, given her previous obstetric history. Her second baby was also bigger than the first, so it was not unlikely that there would be a problem again.

The labour progressed until the second stage, when there was a delay and it appeared that the baby was stuck.

The midwife on duty, Mona, summoned the GP and when he arrived the baby was in distress. Mona had also called for assistance from the nearest large obstetric unit, but the ambulance was yet to arrive. So the GP tried to deliver the baby with forceps.

The baby's skull was fractured in several places and he was very ill when he arrived at our hospital. His mother had been badly torn internally and needed to go straight to theatre to be stitched up before she haemorrhaged. Sadly, the baby died from his injuries while she was still in the theatre. My colleague Anne and I were newly pregnant at the time and probably more emotional than usual. We sat with Eve and her husband Colin and tried to comfort them, but their grief was so intense that Anne and I simply sobbed along with them.

All the midwives were upset, as they always are when a baby dies. The poor GP was inconsolable. He had made the difficult decision to intervene and done his best, because he feared the baby would die before help arrived. After the parents had got over their initial anger, they forgave him. They understood that his intentions had been good and that human error happens.

But one of the obstetric consultants who heard about the tragedy vowed that she would do everything she could to close the GP unit down. I felt this was unfair, as the biggest mistake that had been made was allowing Eve to book at the unit. I couldn't help thinking of a blunder that this particular consultant had made herself not long before, with a woman who had been in hospital for weeks because her second baby had not been growing well.

The foetal heart monitor was used to assess the baby's condition twice a day. The machine is attached to the mother using two belts around her abdomen and a record of the baby's heart is printed out. One day, the baby's heart rate was reported to the consultant as being unsatisfactory and she made the decision to deliver the baby by caesarean section two days later, on her operating day. But the baby died the following day.

The parents were grief-stricken and angry. They felt they had been badly let down. They instructed solicitors to sue, something that was much less common then than it is now, thirty years later. They were not able to have another baby because of the woman's medical problems. I was thankful that they already had a little girl. I knew it didn't make up for their loss, but it gave them a reason to carry on living.

Anyway, the consultant got her way and the GP unit did close down, so for me the opening of our birth centre was especially touching. The midwives enjoyed working there and we managed to maintain a small, friendly, non-interventionist environment. Everyone was very proud of the unit and staff and locals alike took part in fundraising activities to buy new equipment for the parents-to-be to use.

Unfortunately, our satisfaction was short-lived, because within a couple of years the hospital trust management decided to close it down in another round of cost cutting.

This was a huge disappointment to everyone and meant once again that women would have to travel a greater distance to the nearest hospital. It was also soul-destroying for the midwives who had worked so hard to get the centre up and running and had seen it becoming so successful. Worst of all, it was a complete waste of taxpayers' money, as well as a waste of the money that had been donated by various organisations and businesses in the area.

Still, I am hopeful that one day common sense will prevail and there will once again be birth centres opening around the country. They really are great places to give birth.

18

The End of an Era

At the time of writing, I have now been a midwife for over thirty years and I think I've been very lucky to have had such a wonderful career. There have been so many high-lights, but the best, without doubt, was bringing my own granddaughter into the world. What made it even more exciting was that it wasn't planned!

My son, Edward, and daughter-in-law live in a different area to the one where I work and they decided on a home birth for their second baby. My role during the labour was to collect my grandson and look after him until the baby arrived.

My son telephoned early on a Sunday morning and asked Derek and me to come over. 'There's no rush, so take your time,' he said confidently. Knowing that second babies can come very quickly, I insisted on getting there as soon as possible. When we arrived, it was obvious that labour was very advanced. 'Call the midwife and tell her to come as soon as possible!' I urged my son.

About a week earlier, I had been talking about the imminent arrival with my daughter, Lucy. 'Imagine if the booked midwife didn't turn up and I had to deliver the baby!' I said.

It was supposed to be a joke. I never dreamed it would actually happen . . .

I was right about the second labour being quick. The baby decided it was time to make an appearance and Derek was duly instructed to take our grandson, Harry, to the park. Every delivery is special but I can honestly say that I have never felt such a combination of intense focus and pure excitement at any other birth. If I'd had time in all the rush, I would have pinched myself – it was simply a dream come true. Fortunately, although it was fast, it was a very straightforward delivery and as I caught my new granddaughter, I knew that this was a moment of joy that I would remember forever. What a privilege to be there! By the time the midwife turned up, mum, dad and a very proud grandmother were sitting down and admiring baby Molly. Derek brought Harry back to meet his new sister and, after many tears and a lot of smiles, we left to give the family some time together.

I was still walking on air at the birthday party we went to later. It was for my friend Alison's daughter, whom I had delivered twenty-one years earlier. I couldn't stop telling people about our exciting morning and the new birthday girl. It was a thrilling connection to have with my little granddaughter.

It has also been my privilege to deliver my brother's three children, as well as many friends' babies. It can be difficult when there is an emotional involvement, though. Part of you must stay detached and remain professional so that you can do the job properly; meanwhile another part of you is desperate to behave like a friend or relative and give loving care and support. Of course, you can be similarly split with the pregnant women you have got to know well, but with them it is easier to be dispassionate enough to deal with problems if necessary, whereas there is always the worry that you will miss something important with a friend or relative, simply because it's harder to remain professional when your emotions are all stirred up.

I was delighted to be asked to deliver my brother and sister-in-law's first child at home. My nephew was born in the house where my mother had spent her last days, and I couldn't help thinking about this during the birth. It made me sad to think she would never meet this grandchild. But I reasoned that my mother would have been so happy that he was born in the home where she had lived for most of her married life. There was a lovely sense of continuity about it.

When you reach your fifties, people start to talk about retirement. But how can you retire from a job that has not just been your career, but your life? Many of my colleagues have seemed happy to end their working life and it's been a relief for them to put an end to the stresses and strains of the job. I don't feel quite ready to give up, though. I no longer want to rebel or to be dynamic like some of the younger midwives, which makes me feel like I've come to the end of an era. But I do want to be with mothers and babies and give them and their families help and support. And I still want to teach students how to be good midwives.

Everything about midwifery is different thirty years on. People are more aware of their rights, and litigation in obstetrics is rife. The new compensation culture has had a detrimental effect on midwifery. Midwives have to spend so much time writing notes about everything that is said and done during labour that they actually have very little opportunity to care for and cherish the woman. What's more, they are always thinking about the possibility of ending up in a court of law and having to defend their decision making; student midwives are taught to be vigilant in this area at all times. It's a stressful way to work.

People seem to expect that they will get expert care and exclusive attention in hospital, but this is not always the case. There are often severe shortages of staff and this means that the midwives on duty are left trying to do more than they can realistically cope with. This can cause problems when women and their partners feel neglected, and unhappy with their experience of childbirth; it can have long-term effects on their parenting, relationships and family life.

Thirty years ago, there were more small maternity units; they were coping with fewer women and had more staff. It was accepted that senior midwives were the experts. They guided the junior doctors and collaborated with the senior doctors, so that there was a sense of unity in working for the benefit of the patients, rather than to avoid litigation. This meant that people generally had a good experience and there was far less intervention in their labours.

Nowadays many smaller hospitals and birth centres have closed down and women give birth in large maternity units, where about seventeen babies a day are born and sometimes more than one in four women have a caesarean. The midwives do their best, but how can women get the sort of birth experience they deserve when the sheer numbers passing through the maternity unit turn it into a production line? The whole ethos of birth has changed. It is for these reasons that there is now a shortage of midwives; people just don't want to work in these conditions.

When I reminisce with colleagues, we always talk about how much we enjoyed coming to work and how we worked hard but also had lots of fun. This is no longer true for most midwives. Working in a smaller unit meant that you got to know the patients quite well, especially as the length of stay after the birth used to be eight days, and ten days after a caesarean section. Now they're in and out in no time, discharged to free up a bed as much as for health reasons. It's all about saving money.

Times change of course, and in midwifery, as in every area of life, the profession changes to reflect new social attitudes and new ways of doing things. Some of this feels like progress, but there was often a reason for the old ways. One good example is this question of bed rest after the birth. Although I can understand that women want to be at home with their partners and families, they are not always sufficiently prepared to cope with all that having a new baby entails. When the hospital stay was longer, they were given the time to rest and recover from the birth and the opportunity to talk through their experience with an unhurried, interested midwife. Visiting hours were stricter, which was hard on the fathers but did ensure much-needed peace and quiet. Also, mothers were valued and cared for and shown how to look after a baby, so that they would feel confident when they returned home. Of course, much of it is common sense, but there are little things parents can be shown that can make life so much easier for them.

Women now go home the day after a vaginal birth and on the third day after a caesarean section. Pain relief these days is so effective that friends and family often forget that their loved one has been through a major physical trauma and expect too much from them. It is not unknown for the women themselves to overdo things by going round the supermarket on the way home from hospital! Not a good idea for the woman or baby. For the baby there is the risk of infection and for the mother a risk of haemorrhage. But it is seen as a triumph if women regain their figures and go back to work soon after giving birth. Media coverage of actresses and dynamic businesswomen sends out a message to ordinary mothers that they must lose their baby weight and recover control of their lives within weeks. So women feel they have to try to emulate these celebrities, or else see themselves as failures. Yet in some societies women are cocooned in a loving, extended family when they have given birth and are not allowed to do anything for themselves until they have fully recuperated. We seem to have lost any vestige of this tradition.

After the birth, women used to be visited by a community midwife every day for ten days and sometimes longer. But because of the current shortage of midwives, this is no longer possible; more midwives are needed on the labour ward, the highest risk area, leaving the minimum number to work out in the community. A new mum can expect perhaps three half-hour visits during the first two weeks of a baby's life at home, when the midwife will struggle to give her anything more than the most important information. Mothers having second or subsequent babies may not need many visits, but first-time parents are usually very grateful for support and reassurance. They may also need counselling if they have had a bad experience, and they see the midwife as a liaison between them and the hospital. The adjustment to parenthood is huge and should not be underestimated.

Some people think that having children can repair a rocky marriage, but the reality is that it may break it completely. Some mothers are lucky and have families to help them when they return home. But many people have no-one and struggle to cope with normal family life, while trying to match society's expectations of them. They feel under so much pressure to be back to normal after this huge life-changing experience that they end up with post-natal depression when they fear they are failing.

The number of midwives on the postnatal ward has also diminished over the decades. Dedicated and caring people, they often find that they are not able to give their desired level of care because they have to look after so many women and there are too many demands on their time. One in four women has a caesarean section, so midwifery care becomes post-operative nursing care as well. This means attending to intravenous drips, catheters with urine bags and pain relief, as well as changing and feeding babies. Helping the woman to recover, while looking after the baby and initiating breastfeeding, is time-consuming and impossible to do well if you are caring for a large number of women at the same time. No wonder twenty-first century parents are complaining about their experiences of childbirth. Post-traumatic stress syndrome is now a recognised illness in women who have had a bad childbirth experience and it has a knock-on effect on family life. And of course midwives are leaving the profession in droves because they are so dissatisfied.

What has happened to our beloved NHS? The hospital trusts that are severely in debt seem to make cuts in all the wrong places. There are too many managers and adminis-trators and too many different departments within the Trust, all with unfathomable titles and names. For exam-ple, why do they need a Director of Planning, a Director of Delivery, a Director of Workforce, a Director of Partnerships, and a Director of Corporate Affairs, to name but a few? And how many members of staff are employed by each of these departments?

When I was helping to set up our birth centre, I had an insight into the work of some of these departments and saw first-hand all the meetings that are held, where noth-ing is achieved except establishing the date for the next meeting! Most administrators I've met seem totally oblivi-ous to the plight of the midwives on the wards. There may be just two staff working on the postnatal ward, trying to look after thirty-two women and their babies. They may be struggling because one colleague is off sick and another has been drafted to the delivery suite to help out. The administrators don't see the situation as their problem, but surely the Trust's first duty is to the welfare of its patients and staff?

Money gets transferred from one NHS organisation to

another, creating numerous jobs where people are simply pushing paper around. I understand this is known as the 'market approach', but it means less money for the staff on the ground caring for the patients, which has to be wrong. What's more, each trust should have its own in-house staff to provide cleaning and food services. Now that these jobs are put out to tender, it is very difficult to police the workers, which may partly explain the spread of hospital-acquired infection.

This madness has even spread to the wards in hospital, where modern matrons are multiplying. Unlike the old-fashioned matron, who appeared to run the entire hospital single-handedly, these professionals are in charge of various areas. They are often promoted because of their length of service, not because they are good managers and leaders. Sometimes the promotion goes to their heads and they become autocratic and bullying. It seems to me that they are mostly to be found in their offices, drawing up policies and protocols and attending meetings with each other to chew over their latest set of directives. The endless documents they produce seem designed to overrule common sense, kindness and compassion and stifle creativity and innovation. A midwife can be suspended or even dismissed for not adhering to hospital policy, even if it is detrimental to the wellbeing of the patient.

Thankfully, there are still many wonderful midwives practising within the NHS, because the profession will always attract caring, compassionate people who want to play a vital part in the miracle of birth.

*   *   *

Whatever the NHS's problems, I've adored my job for decades and retirement still feels like a big step. That said, I think my husband will be pleased when he no longer gets woken up in the early hours by the phone ringing off the hook. Partners of midwives are special. They do a lot of childcare and never know if they will get a meal cooked for them – or whether their partner will even come home at all! It is normal for a community midwife to work a ten-hour shift, be called to a woman in labour and not to finish work until twenty-four hours after first leaving home. Then there are the Christmases and Easters when partners will be celebrating on their own or visiting their parents for hearty meals and help with children. Still, Derek now has an extensive knowledge of childbirth and is proud to be 'The Pregnancy Advisor' at his place of work!

Another reason for contemplating retirement is that my hearing is deteriorating. I explain my difficulties to the women in my care and they are always very supportive. However, deafness is such a hidden disability that people forget you are affected. It is quite irksome to have to constantly remind people to face me so that I can lip-read and study their body language to help me understand what they're saying. Also, I can't hear whispering, people speaking from down a corridor, telephone callers with strong accents and, most importantly, gossip between colleagues when several people are talking at once.

'You're wearing hearing aids, so why can't you hear?' one manager asked.

'Would you expect someone with a prosthetic leg to be

able to run a marathon?' I replied. Such ignorance in the medical profession is unforgivable.

I don't wish to sound self-pitying as I do actually see the funny side of life with a hearing impairment. I was running an antenatal clinic at one of the local surgeries one day when a woman arrived having contractions. I think she wanted confirmation that she was actually in labour before getting to the hospital where she was booked in. I briefly examined her and confirmed that she was definitely going to have the baby that afternoon. I was worried that she wouldn't have time to call her partner home from work to collect her, so I asked the surgery receptionist to call an ambulance, thinking that I could get her partner to meet her at the hospital.

While speaking to ambulance control the receptionist called over to me and asked the woman's name . . . or so I thought.

'Is it Cheryl Fletcher?'

'No, that's not her name,' I replied, not wishing to divulge it in front of the other patients.

But she just repeated, 'Cheryl Fletcher?'

And again I said, 'No it's not!'

Then another receptionist stepped in and said, 'Agnes, she is asking if you require a chair or stretcher!!!'

Of course I turned bright red. We all laughed when I recounted the tale to the family that evening at home. Now whenever I mishear and make a daft comment or give a funny answer to their questions, they raise their eyebrows at each other. 'Mum's doing a Cheryl Fletcher!'

Another time, a young woman with a strong Welsh

accent came to the antenatal clinic I was running. After the formalities I asked if she had any questions. 'I'm fat,' she confided. 'Is that a problem, do you think?'

I was confused, as she didn't look fat to me, so I thought she was just being extra sensitive about her changing body. 'No, that's not a problem at all,' I reassured her.

She smiled and happily left the surgery. As I browsed through her medical notes later, I suddenly saw the words 'works as a vet' and realised that I had misheard her because of her strong accent. What she had said to me was not 'I'm fat' but 'I'm a vet'! She must have thought I was incompetent, as there are definitely things to watch out for when you are pregnant and working with animals. She obviously knew this and wanted confirmation. Oh dear, another deaf-as-a-doughnut moment!

So retirement beckons, but I can't imagine a life without caring for people, so I will probably have to do some voluntary work after having a rest and gathering my thoughts for a while. When I look back and consider the little girl I once was, so determined to be a nurse and then a midwife, and I think of all the obstacles and hard graft it took to get there, I can see that I have been very lucky to have worked virtually all my life at something I passionately believed was important. I still believe that midwives are unsung heroines, that the comfort they give can literally change a woman's life, as it once did mine. There's no doubt in my mind that their skills can mean the difference between life and death.

One thing is for sure, I will never forget all the women

and their babies whose stories I have told. I consider myself very privileged indeed to have been a part of their lives and shared such intimate times with them. However much I managed to give them, it was far outweighed by the joy and satisfaction they gave me in return.

Acknowledgements

Firstly, thank you to Ajda Vucicevic for her belief in me. Thank you also to Fenella Bates and her team at Hodder for their help and encouragement. Thank you to Rebecca Cripps for her contribution.

Lastly, thank you to my husband for his love and support, and endless cups of tea!